Audrey Borden

The History
of Gay People
in Alcoholics Anonymous
From the Beginning

*Pre-publication
REVIEWS,
COMMENTARIES,
EVALUATIONS . . .*

"This volume fills in a previously missing chapter in the history of addiction recovery in America. Well-researched and well-written, the book's strength lies in the interviews that allow Borden to weave the personal stories of individuals into a larger story of the history of recovery among gay Americans. These same stories also reveal fascinating details about the history of Alcoholics Anonymous and the history of the gay community in America."

William L. White
Author, *Slaying the Dragon: The History of Addiction Treatment and Recovery in America*

"This groundbreaking book about an important but little-known part of the history of Alcoholics Anonymous belongs on the shelves of every alcoholic and addict, straight or gay. Counselors, clinicians, clergy, and their teachers will find it an invaluable resource. Audrey Borden has done a magnificent job of interweaving over thirty fascinating interviews of influential LGBT AAs and their contributions, spanning fifty years to the present, with factual information about the gradual acceptance by Alcoholics Anonymous itself. I wish my husband and I had had this excellent account ourselves when we wrote our own book about Marty Mann, one of AA's earliest leaders."

Rev. Sally Brown, MS, MDiv
Board Certified Clinical Chaplain (retired), United Church of Christ; Co-Author of *A Biography of Mrs. Marty Mann: The First Lady of Alcoholics Anonymous*

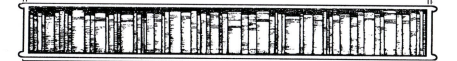

More pre-publication
REVIEWS, COMMENTARIES, EVALUATIONS . . .

"This work addresses an important and largely ignored topic—gays and lesbians in Alcoholics Anonymous—through fascinating accounts from gays and lesbians in San Francisco, Los Angeles, and New York who have been sober for many years and have lived through the changes in attitudes and treatment of gays and lesbians in the larger society and culture and within AA. This fascinating book is an important first step in chronicling and understanding the experiences of gays and lesbians in AA and is a window into the ways in which AA is like and unlike the larger society. Borden covers how the Third Tradition, which was developed in the 1940s, opened AA to all who suffered from their drinking. She sensitively deals with the pros and cons of separate gay/lesbian meetings and the attitudes of many that gays and lesbians should also be welcome and feel comfortable in general AA meetings. As in the larger society, there were many closeted gay meetings in the 1950s known only by word of mouth, but by the 1970s' era of advocacy, this began to change, with open struggles found in various communities. As one narrator summarized, while AA had its biases and limitations in welcoming gays and lesbians, AA was also more accepting and less prejudicial than the larger society."

Thomasina Borkmman, PhD
Professor Emerita of Sociology,
George Mason University, Fairfax, VA

"The author lets a number of people speak in their own voices, from their own powerful and moving experiences. These are voices that have not been heard enough over the past years. I was very impressed and edified by the quality of hope, faith, and service that they point to and draw from. This book sheds light on a long-neglected treasure trove, and I am grateful that it is now available to fellow searchers and seekers; it is useful and hopeful and most welcome. The men and women interviewed here are wonderful to meet, and wonderful to listen to."

Fr. Thomas Weston, S. J.
Oakland, CA

The Haworth Press
New York

The History
of Gay People
in Alcoholics Anonymous
From the Beginning

HAWORTH SERIES IN FAMILY AND CONSUMER ISSUES IN HEALTH
F. Bruce Carruth, PhD
Senior Editor

Addicted and Mentally Ill: Stories of Courage, Hope, and Empowerment by Carol Bucciarelli

The History of Gay People in Alcoholics Anonymous: From the Beginning by Audrey Borden

The History of Gay People in Alcoholics Anonymous

From the Beginning

Audrey Borden

The Haworth Press
New York

For more information on this book or to order, visit
http://www.haworthpress.com/store/product.asp?sku=5699

or call 1-800-HAWORTH (800-429-6784) in the United States and Canada
or (607) 722-5857 outside the United States and Canada

or contact orders@HaworthPress.com

Published by

The Haworth Press, Inc., 10 Alice Street, Binghamton, NY 13904-1580.

PUBLISHER'S NOTE
The development, preparation, and publication of this work has been undertaken with great care. However, the Publisher, employees, editors, and agents of The Haworth Press are not responsible for any errors contained herein or for consequences that may ensue from use of materials or information contained in this work. The Haworth Press is committed to the dissemination of ideas and information according to the highest standards of intellectual freedom and the free exchange of ideas. Statements made and opinions expressed in this publication do not necessarily reflect the views of the Publisher, Directors, management, or staff of The Haworth Press, Inc., or an endorsement by them.

Cover design by Marylouise Doyle.

Library of Congress Cataloging-in-Publication Data

Borden, Audrey.
    The history of gay people in Alcoholics Anonymous : from the beginning / Audrey Borden.
    p. cm.
    Includes bibliographical references and index.
    ISBN: 978-0-7890-3038-2 (hard : alk. paper)
    ISBN: 978-0-7890-3039-9 (soft : alk. paper)
    1. Gays—Alcohol use—United States—History. 2. Alcoholics—Rehabilitation—United States. 3. Recovering alcoholics—United States. 4. Alcoholics Anonymous—History. I. Title.
HV5139.B67 2007
362.292'86086642—dc22
                                                                            2006037370

To the recovering community

ABOUT THE AUTHOR

Audrey Borden has been writing for many years, primarily for the software industry, and has been involved with the recovering community in the San Francisco Bay Area since the early 1980s. She has a bachelor's degree in geography from Portland State University in Oregon. She lives with her wife and daughter in Marin County, California.

CONTENTS

Preface

"Here," said my mother-in-law, holding out a book, "I thought you might like to read this."

"Um, sure, thanks," I said, taking it from her, hoping I didn't sound too disinterested. I glanced at the title, *Mrs. Marty Mann: The First Lady of Alcoholics Anonymous,* and started flipping through it absentmindedly from the back until I came to a collection of old photographs. There I saw something that made me sit bolt upright on the sofa. There was an elegant portrait of Mrs. Mann and her life partner Priscilla Peck.

Life partner?

Marty Mann—founder of the National Council on Alcoholism, friend and colleague of Alcoholics Anonymous (AA) cofounder Bill Wilson since AA's early days in New York, the woman who opened AA's doors to thousands of alcoholics in the 1940s and 1950s—was a lesbian? Now, that got my attention! I took that book home and read it cover to cover.

When I'd finished, I went to the living room and took an old audiotape out of a drawer, a cherished recording of a talk given by an AA member named Barry L. at a convention in 1985. I dropped *The Gay Origins of AA's Third Tradition* into the tape player and settled back for another hour of AA history.

Although I'd heard Barry's tape many times before, I noticed that this time something was different and it took me a while to figure out what it was. I realized that I knew the names and stories of many of the people Barry referred to anonymously in his talk. Of course! One of the two "homosexual persons" he met in AA was Marty. And the more I listened, the clearer it became that my ideas about being gay in AA in the 1940s and 1950s were all wrong. Marty and Barry weren't the lonely, isolated gay people I'd imagined them to be, far from it. Their lives and those of many early AA members, including Bill Wil-

The History of Gay People in Alcoholics Anonymous
Published by The Haworth Press, Inc., 2007. All rights reserved.
doi:10.1300/5699_a

son and his wife, Al-Anon cofounder Lois Wilson, were interconnected.

And suddenly, there stood before me a long line of gay people in AA, stretching back from present-day California to 1937, to Akron, Ohio, to the night a gay man summoned all his courage and asked if *he* would be allowed to join Alcoholics Anonymous. Gay people had always been a part of AA! I vowed to find them, and to tell their story.

I began reading everything I could find on alcoholism, gay history, and Alcoholics Anonymous. I read histories, biographies, and memoirs. I learned about the challenges of writing about historic people who had been gay.[1] I lurked in libraries and sifted through databases filled with research papers on an astonishing array of alcohol-related topics, and I quickly learned two things:

1. Books about alcoholism rarely mention gay people.
2. Books about gay people rarely mention alcoholism.

The first fact didn't surprise me—studies of alcoholics focus overwhelmingly on white heterosexual males—but the second one did, given the number of books that discuss the importance of bars in gay history and their role in the development of gay communities. Even detailed studies of early bar communities bypassed the role alcohol may have played in those groups (Kennedy and Davis 1994; Beemyn 1997). I was also saddened that I was able to find only a single document on the topic of long-term sobriety. In fact, the *Alcohol and Other Drug Thesaurus: A Guide to Concepts and Terminology in Substance Abuse and Addiction,* an annotated listing of more than 11,000 concepts spanning the addiction field and organized by subject, had no listing for "Long-Term Sobriety."

When I contacted Sally and David Brown, the authors of Marty Mann's biography, they were delighted to hear from me and gave me a list of people I ought to call. One of them, George M., e-mailed an introduction on my behalf to the people on the Browns' list that he knew, and to several more as well. And so it went—each person I talked to gave me more people to contact.

It wasn't long before I realized that most of the people on my growing list of contacts had entered AA in New York, San Francisco, or Los Angeles. With assistance from the International Advisory Council of Homosexual Men and Women, I was able to locate people who'd entered AA far away from the cities on the East and West Coasts with established gay communities. Unfortunately, my efforts to find people of color with long-term sobriety were less successful.

I wanted to conduct face-to-face interviews with as many people as possible, but I knew that in most cases I'd have to rely on the telephone. Although I'd initially viewed this as a limitation, I discovered that interviewing by phone had some unforeseen advantages. One was the greater level of anonymity it provided, and because the narrators and I spoke at length without visual cues, I found the phone helped reduce some of the social awkwardness that can arise when people have different cultural, ethnic, generational, and class backgrounds.

In keeping with AA's tradition of anonymity, only the first name and last initial of identified AA members appear in this book. Some narrators asked to appear under a pseudonym, and in cases where the details of someone's story made it possible to identify that person, I asked the narrator to select a pseudonym I could use in place of his or her name and initial. Following the practice of leaving one's professional, political, and religious affiliations out of AA-related discussions, I limited my questions in those areas to a few basic facts.

One last issue related to anonymity dogged my conscience. My goal was to document—and to celebrate—the contributions of gay and lesbian people in AA. But early on in the interview process, a former AA trustee raised a red flag: Wouldn't this approach place some AA members above others in the reader's eyes? What about AA's tradition of selfless service to other alcoholics? Finally, after much deliberation and some long talks with friends in AA, I was reminded that while AA members are anonymous, AA's message is not. In other words, as long as I focused on what someone had done, rather than on *who* had done it, I'd be upholding AA's Twelfth Tradition in the broadest possible sense. I would document how individuals' actions had allowed the spirit of AA to work through them.

Words and Silence

Narrative analysis shows us how language, structure, and context convey meaning in a story. Historians study what has been said and written in the past, but I often found myself in the curious position of studying what hadn't been said and what hadn't been written.

When I first began interviewing people, I naively thought they would use words and phrases I'd find old-fashioned, for example, that a narrator might say, "I'm a homosexual," rather than, "I'm a lesbian" or "I'm gay." This was never the case. Although other generational and culturally based issues arose, terminology was never a problem. But I did find a problem when I started transcribing the interviews, *a very big problem.*

As I transcribed the interviews, when approaching a critical passage, such as the point where the narrator talked about his or her experience of being gay, I noticed that key words and phrases were missing—words such as "gay," "lesbian," "homosexual," and "queer." It was as if they'd been erased from the tape. Instead, there would be a subtle pause, a gap, where I was expected to fill in the words they'd left unspoken. Reviewing my experience of each interview, I recalled that it was at those moments that I'd felt I knew *exactly* what the narrator was trying to say. The communication had been so seamless that it wasn't until I transferred the spoken words to paper that I had any awareness that any words were missing.

How was I to transcribe all those missing words? At first, I tried filling in the blanks by guessing, and calling people back to find out if I had guessed correctly—what an ineffective, labor-intensive way to complete an interview. But then I found that the most effective way of conveying the narrator's intent, and his or her experience of telling the story, was to describe the silence. For example, here is how I transcribed this passage from Barry L.'s presentation, *The Gay Origins of the Third Tradition:*

> I remember that I was a little bit late finding out about some *[pausing, and clearing his throat]* . . . sex matters. I was actually in my teens when I discovered that *[cough]*—I went into show business.

And now, with great pleasure, I give you *The History of Gay People in Alcoholics Anonymous: From the Beginning,* a book where the words "alcoholism," "homosexual," "recovery," "lesbian," and "queer" comfortably occupy the same page. I hope reading it is as illuminating an experience for you as writing it has been for me.

Acknowledgments

Among the many people who supported this project, I'd like to especially thank archivist Rob M. at the California Northern Coastal Area AA Archives and the staff at the AA Archives in New York; the Living Sober Conference's planning committees, the GLBT Historical Society, and the central AA office in San Francisco; the International Advisory Council of Homosexual Men and Women in Alcoholics Anonymous; and the Alcohol Research Group Library in Berkeley.

The librarians at the Belvedere-Tiburon library, especially Abbot Chambers and the others on the reference desk who located texts for me, were invaluable. Caroline Pincus (the Book Midwife), and Bruce Carruth at The Haworth Press, both provided valuable editing direction. The *AA Grapevine* Digital Archive and members of the AA History Lovers e-mail list continue to be a source of information and inspiration.

A special thanks to my friends Mary Bishop and Beverly Wagstaff for their support. Thanks to Jane H. for the copy of *Mrs. Marty Mann: The First Lady of Alcoholics Anonymous* and a place to work. And finally, my thanks to my wife Catherine, for her encouragement, patience, and good advice.

Excerpts from the workshop, Gays in AA: A Part Of or Apart From?, recorded at the Seventh International AA Convention in New Orleans, 1980, appear with the permission of the Freeman Company, Dallas, Texas.

Excerpts from "Communication and Culture": Copyright © The AA Grapevine, Inc. (September 1993). Reprinted with permission. Permission to reprint The AA Grapevine, Inc., copyrighted material in this publication does not in any way imply affiliation with or endorsement by Alcoholics Anonymous or The AA Grapevine, Inc.

The History of Gay People in Alcoholics Anonymous
Published by The Haworth Press, Inc., 2007. All rights reserved.
doi:10.1300/5699_b

PART I:
FROM THE BEGINNING,
1935-1970

Chapter 1

The Recovering Gay Community

Introduction

Not so very long ago, it was against the law for homosexuals to gather in public. Books and plays portraying homosexuality as anything other than a vice, a sin, or an illness were ruled obscene and banned. But if you were gay, there was a place you could go to find other gay people: you could go to a bar. Most gay bars were windowless dives, where patrons endured inflated prices, police harassment, arrest, and assault by thugs entering and leaving these establishments. But oh! Once inside, you could feel it, that sense of connection, of community, of *belonging* somewhere.

But starting in the early 1940s in New York City, a small group of gay men and women were having a very different experience of being together. In well-lit public venues, in meeting halls where people talked frankly about their lives, gay people began to find one another in Alcoholics Anonymous (AA). They were the first men and women to belong to what has now become an international fellowship of thousands of gay, lesbian, bisexual, and transgender (GLBT) people in AA, Al-Anon, Narcotics Anonymous, and other twelve-step programs, known collectively as the gay recovering community.

Today, there are roughly 1,800 gay AA meetings a week in the United States, and gay AA groups meet in over sixty foreign cities.[1] But few people outside this diverse community are aware of these groups or the tremendous good they do. Because despite our modern understanding of alcoholism as a disease, and a growing acceptance of gay people in our society, stigmas against homosexuality and alco-

The History of Gay People in Alcoholics Anonymous
Published by The Haworth Press, Inc., 2007. All rights reserved.
doi:10.1300/5699_01

3

holism remain strong. Raise either topic in a casual conversation, and you'll find that most people quickly grow uneasy.

AA and Al-Anon, for families and friends of alcoholics, provide a supportive environment for people healing from alcoholism. Millions of families have been torn apart by the disease, and as it maintains its grip on a steady 8 percent of the U.S. population, millions more will be affected in the coming decade.

Here are some recent statistics on alcoholism and drug addiction from the U.S. Department of Health and Human Services, the National Council on Alcoholism and Drug Dependence, and the *Encyclopedia of Public Health:*

- Roughly fourteen million Americans meet the diagnostic criteria for alcohol abuse or alcoholism. Twenty-three million Americans suffer from substance abuse addiction.
- About 100,000 U.S. deaths are attributed to alcohol abuse each year. Alcohol-related deaths occur from cancer, cirrhosis of the liver, pancreatitis, motor vehicle crashes, falls, drowning, suicide, and homicide. Worldwide 750,000 deaths are attributed to alcohol use each year.
- More than half of all American adults have a close family member who has or has had alcoholism. Approximately one in four children under the age of eighteen is exposed to alcohol abuse or alcohol dependence in the family. More than nine million children live with a parent dependent on alcohol and/or illicit drugs.
- One-quarter of all U.S. emergency room admissions, one-third of all suicides, and over half of all homicides and incidents of domestic violence are alcohol-related.
- Untreated addiction costs America $400 billion per year. It is six times more expensive than is America's number one killer, heart disease ($133.2 billion per year), six times more expensive than diabetes ($130 billion per year), and four times more expensive than cancer ($96.1 billion per year).

Table 1.1 offers some numbers from the other side of the scoreboard. AA does not keep membership records, so the numbers in Table 1.1 are not a tally of the people who consider themselves AA members, but they do provide an overview of AA membership.

TABLE 1.1. AA Membership

AA Membership, 2004	Groups	Members
United States	52,651	1,184,979
Canada	4,872	95,984
Correctional Facilities	2,562	66,576
Internationalists (Seagoing)		70
Lone Members		204
Overseas	44,425	716,453
Total Members		2,076,935
Total Groups	105,294	

Source: Alcoholics Anonymous, 2005.

An analysis of the responses to AA's 2004 triennial membership survey in the United States and Canada showed that 50 percent had over five years sobriety, 26 percent had less than one year sobriety, and 50 percent had five years or less. The average length of sobriety was over eight years. Among the 7,500 respondents, 65 percent were men, 35 percent were women, 89.1 percent were white, 4.4 percent were Hispanic, 3.2 percent were black, 1.8 percent were Native American, and 1.5 percent were Asian and "others" (Alcoholics Anonymous 2004 Membership Survey 2005). AA does not currently include a question about sexual orientation on the survey, so I cannot offer any data on the number of AA members who identify as GLBT.

About the Chapters Ahead

This book is organized roughly in chronological and then geographical order. In Chapter 2, Barry L. provides a rich description of what was happening in New York AA in the 1940s and describes key events in gay AA history that I discuss later in detail. Chapter 3 gives an overview of the many treatments for homosexuality and alcoholism, and some of the parallels between the ways gay people and alcoholics were treated in the twentieth century. In Chapter 4, you'll meet five AA members who came into AA in the 1940s and 1950s.

In Chapter 5, I provide an overview of the different kinds of AA meetings and how group directories are used to find them. This chapter includes a tribute to gay AA group names. In Chapter 6, Nancy T.

talks about her role in getting information about AA to the gay community, when AA itself could not. Chapter 7 discusses "special purpose" groups in AA and their role in the debate over gay groups in Alcoholics Anonymous. It closes with John W.'s account of the events at the historic 1974 General Service Conference, and his efforts to bring black AA members into the all-white AA service structure in Washington DC.

In Part II, you'll meet AA members from around the country who entered AA between 1961 and 1981, including cofounders of the first gay meetings, and people who got sober in rural communities and small towns. You'll hear from distinguished professionals in the addiction field, and learn the history of AA's pamphlet for gay and lesbian alcoholics. I conclude with answers to some of the questions I set out to answer when I began my research, and my thoughts on *what it all means.*

Timeline of Key Events, 1937-1990

The following tables provide an overview of some key events in gay AA history.

TABLE 1.2. Timeline of Key Events, 1937-1967

Year	Key Events
1937	A gay man goes to see AA cofounder Robert Smith in Akron. He tells him he's a homosexual and asks if he can join AA.
1939	First printing of AA's main text, *Alcoholics Anonymous.* Marty M. becomes the first female alcoholic (and the first lesbian) in the first AA group in New York, which meets weekly at the Wilson's home in Brooklyn. Not long afterward Marty's partner Priscilla P. joins AA. Marty and Priscilla are among the first women to achieve long-term sobriety in AA.
1944	After discussing the idea with Bill Wilson, in New York, an AA member named Lois K. meets with Priscilla and Marty to discuss publishing an AA magazine.
1945	First issue of the *AA Grapevine* published. Its six founding members are Lois K., Priscilla P., Marty M., Chase H., Maeve S., Bud T., and Kay M.
1949	An AA group for homosexual alcoholics begins meeting in a men's rooming house in Boston on Beacon Hill.
1950	AA formally adopts the Twelve Traditions, though different groups continue to have widely varying requirements for membership. In New York City gay and lesbian AA members have already developed a growing network.

TABLE 1.2 *(continued)*

Year	Key Events
1954	Marty M. founds the National Council on Alcoholism.
1957	Known among their members as "the Red Door" and "the Saturday Night Follies," two New York meetings have become gay groups, though this is not indicated anywhere in print.
1965	Across the country in San Francisco, the Telegraph Hill Group and the Under 35 Group in North Beach have established local reputations as groups with many gay members.
1967	The American Medical Association (AMA) passes a resolution formally recognizing alcoholism as a disease.

TABLE 1.3. Timeline of Key Events, 1968-1974

Year	Key Events
1968	The first AA group for gay alcoholics begins meeting in a church on Fell Street in San Francisco.
1969	Alcoholics Together, the first gay AA group in Los Angeles, is founded. In New York men and women corralled in a police raid on a gay bar fight back, sparking what will become known as the Stonewall Rebellion.
1970	Gay groups in California start trying to register with the AA General Service Office (GSO) in New York. Questions arise at GSO about whether or not AA groups for homosexuals should appear in the *World Directory,* GSO's directory of registered AA groups.
1971	The Gay Group, the first in Washington DC, is founded.
1972	The New Group, the first gay AA group in New York City, is founded.
1973	The American Psychiatric Association removes homosexuality from its *Diagnostic and Statistical Manual of Mental Disorders.*
	The pamphlet *The Homosexual Alcoholic: A.A.'s Message of Hope to Gay Men & Women* is printed in Washington DC.
	The issue of listing gay groups in the *World Directory* is brought to the General Service Conference by the General Service Office staff. Strong opinions surface on both sides of the issue.
1974	After a long and heated debate, the members of the General Service Conference vote to include groups for homosexuals in the *World Directory.* AA offices in a few cities begin including gay meetings in their local directories.
	Along with copies of *The Homosexual Alcoholic,* Nancy T. begins distributing a rapidly expanding directory of gay AA groups in the United States and abroad.

TABLE 1.4. Timeline of Key Events, 1975-1990

Year	Key Events
1975	An impromptu gathering of gay men at the International AA Convention in Denver becomes an unofficial Gay Hospitality Suite. Round-the-clock meetings are translated spontaneously into several languages to a standing-room-only crowd.
	Number of U.S. cities with a gay AA group in 1975: **7**
1976	The first conference for the gay members of AA and Al-Anon takes place in San Francisco. Notice of the event appears in the calendar of the *AA Grapevine.* First publication of AA's pamphlet *Do You Think You're Different?*
1977	Cade W. and Nancy T. give the first of three annual talks on issues affecting gay and lesbian alcoholics to students at the Rutgers Summer School of Alcohol Studies.
1979	The National Association of Lesbian and Gay Addiction Professionals is founded.
	Number of U.S. cities with a gay AA group in 1979: **86**
1980	Workshops for gay and lesbian alcoholics appear on the program at the seventh International AA Convention in New Orleans. The location of a Gay Hospitality Suite is announced from the main stage.
1981	The International Advisory Council of Homosexual Men and Women in Alcoholics Anonymous is founded. The need for a pamphlet for gay alcoholics is raised again at the General Service Conference.
	Number of U.S. cities with a gay AA group in 1981: **156**
1984	The General Service Conference votes not to publish a pamphlet for gay and lesbian alcoholics.
1985	Barry L. gives a talk on the gay origins of AA's Third Tradition at the International AA Convention in Montreal, Canada.
	Number of U.S. cities with a gay AA group in 1985: **227**
1989	Publication of the pamphlet *A.A. and the Gay/Lesbian Alcoholic.*
1990	Number of U.S. cities with a gay AA group in 1990: **311**

Chapter 2

Barry L. and the Gay Origins of AA's Third Tradition

Introduction

I was visiting Minnesota in the summer of 1986 when a friend invited me to join her at the Twin Cities Roundup, a gay Alcoholics Anonymous (AA) conference in Minneapolis/St. Paul. In the meetings and workshops I attended there, and afterward in the halls, I heard people talking about the AA speaker they'd heard the year before, a man named Barry L. Everyone was so taken with this Barry fellow that I purchased his tape just to see what all the fuss was about. And when I got home to San Francisco, I unpacked my bags, put the tape in a drawer, and promptly forgot about it.

When I finally listened to it nearly a year later, I was beside myself. It was amazing. History had never felt so vivid to me, so alive. In addition to his stunning presentation of Bill Wilson telling the history of the Third Tradition, Barry gave firsthand accounts of the controversy over the inclusion of gay groups in AA's directory, and Bill Wilson's unwavering support of gay alcoholics. Barry's description of Hank P.'s last-minute additions to *Alcoholics Anonymous* gave me chills.

I started telling people about the tape and a few of them even agreed to listen to it. Until one day, when I went to my tape drawer to lend it to someone, I discovered that whomever I'd lent it to last had not returned it. It was gone, and eventually I accepted that it was gone for good. Years went by until, sometime in the mid-1990s, I found myself using a little software program called Gopher.

The History of Gay People in Alcoholics Anonymous
Published by The Haworth Press, Inc., 2007. All rights reserved.
doi:10.1300/5699_02

"What a funny name!" I thought. "Wait a minute, wasn't that the name of the outfit that made Barry's tape? The 'Gopher State' Tape Library?" I decided to try to track down another copy. I sent them a letter describing Barry's talk and a check for what I guessed was an appropriate amount for the tape, but when months, and then a year, went by with no response, I gave up. Then one day, I found a small bubble-wrapped envelope in my mailbox. The Gopher State had come through and Barry was back. And this time after listening to the tape once more, I put it away and swore I'd never share it with anyone again.

Following his presentation in Minnesota, Barry traveled to Montreal, Canada, where he gave the same talk the following weekend to an audience of over 1,000 at AA's eighth International Convention. I listened to a recording of that presentation and found I liked the one at the Twin Cities Roundup much better. It's more intimate, more of a conversation than a presentation. When I hear it, I picture the old brick high school where I attended the 1986 conference. I see Barry at the podium in the small auditorium that doubled as a gym, and his audience on the edges of their wooden folding chairs. I feel like I'm there, and it is my honor and privilege to bring you there, too.

Barry was a master storyteller. He could deliver a series of seemingly off-hand remarks that would leave the audience doubled over with laughter. In an effort to convey the feeling of dialogue rather than monologue, and Barry's impeccable delivery, I've included the audience's response in my transcription. In the interest of space, I've edited out some of the less relevant (though very funny) stories that Barry told that night. Of course, the best way to experience Barry's talk is to order the tape for yourself.[1]

Unfortunately, I was unable to discover more about Barry than what he shares about himself on the recording. I did learn that he and his partner of twenty-six years, Spencer B., a longtime member of Al-Anon, lived together in New York, where they were active in their respective programs for many years. In addition to the AA literature he describes in his talk, Barry also wrote Al-Anon's *Lois Remembers: Memoirs of the Co-Founder of Al-Anon and Wife of the Co-Founder of Alcoholics Anonymous,* and coauthored several articles about alcoholism and AA for the scientific community.[2] He was also a regular contributor to the *AA Grapevine* and to *Box 451,* AA's service newsletter.

I did discover that Spencer held the distinction of being the first person in New York, and perhaps the world, to become ill with what would later be identified as AIDS. When Spencer was first hospitalized, none of the specialists he and Barry visited could tell them what was making him so sick; the doctors were as mystified as they were. A small color photograph of the two men appears in the book *Becoming Visible: An Illustrated History of Lesbian and Gay Life in Twentieth-Century America* (McGarry and Wasserman 1998), along with a copy of the letter Barry wrote to their friends when Spencer was first released from the hospital in June 1981, expressing gratitude for their support during his baffling illness.

Dear Friend,

All the personal notes of thanks we wish to write would take months. But we want no one to go that long without knowing of our gratitude. So, this quick copy information-dissemination method is being used for now.

Your many wonderful visits, the month Spencer was in the hospital, your beautiful bouquets, your prayers, cheery cards, treats, telephone calls, and inquiries surely deserve a large share of the credit for his so-far recovery, and both of us thank you profoundly.

After exactly four weeks (scads of yukky tests, two diagnoses: Kaposi cancer, and lobar pneumonia; lots of antibiotics and one chemotherapy session), St. Vincent's dehospitalized SBB Monday June 22, and he says it is great to be at home. Undisturbed sleep!

Medication continues, but there has been practically no fever since coming home, he is again eating solid foods, and has gained some pounds. The cough is receding and the voice is returning.

He hates the weakness, but of course, a long slow convalescence is ahead, plus more chemotherapy. (Does anybody have experience to share about turning excruciatingly dull, maddeningly slow recuperation into magic time?) This will take far more guts and patience than BL thinks *he* could manage.

We hope you will come have tea with us and boost our recovery further some time soon. We'll be in touch.

With love,
Barry L. and Spencer B.

Spencer died in 1982. Three years later, a few weeks after making this historic presentation, Barry L. passed away, in July 1985. I believe he would be delighted to know that you are about to hear it.

"The Gay Origins of the Third Tradition," Excerpts from a Talk by Barry L. at the Twin Cities Roundup, Minneapolis, Minnesota, June 1985

[As Barry approaches the podium, the audience gives him a warm round of applause. As it slowly subsides, he begins.]

It certainly wasn't like this in [AA in] 1945! *[Cheers and laughter]* I was spiritually dead in 1945. Isn't it great to be spiritually alive in '85? Before I forget, I want to thank the committee for the marvelous hospitality. I just love being at this kind of AA meeting—and there haven't been this kind of AA meeting all these years—where I get to see all my tomboy sisters and sissy brothers.

I'm not going to talk about my drinking for several reasons; one is it is so damn boring. We've all heard drunkalogues, you'll hear a lot of them, and they're very important. I try to tell them; I make myself do it at least twice a year because I think it's good to keep that memory green. But I think there is something more important for me to do here tonight.

I want to talk primarily about our Third Tradition and its history, as it has affected me personally, and what I've witnessed in AA from a particular point of view. This is simply one person's viewpoint. None of us, as all of you know, speaks for AA as a whole.

I think the Third Tradition is about people who are not connected, who have felt for a long time that they didn't belong. Who felt alienated, who felt different, one way or another. Whether we actually were or not is unimportant; we felt alienated, isolated, and ostracized. We felt different and outside.

When I was a kid growing up in Texas, I ran away from home a lot. It's an easy picture for me to remember because I was barefoot, I had on bib overalls, and I probably had a bandanna handkerchief with some food in it. I was also a sissy and a 'fraidy cat, so I would never go very far; I always got home by nightfall.

I was not trying to escape from anything, because I had no reason to escape; I was trying to get *in* somewhere. I was trying to find the place where I would feel I really belonged. And for many years after I was—I started to say a grown person, well, I was tall, anyhow—taller—I kept thinking, *I was born in the wrong century; that's what's the matter with me.* And then I would take another drink.

I was not running away from home because I was unloved. I was loved at home. I was running away from home to find someplace I belonged. And I remember that I was a little bit late finding out about some *[pausing and clearing his throat]* . . . sex matters. I was actually in my teens when I discovered that *[cough]*—I went into show business. *[Laughter]* And I discovered in show business—this was never discussed at home—that when most adults engaged in sexual activity they had partners! *[Laughter]* And I thought that was a very jolly idea! *[More laughter]* I wondered why I hadn't thought of it myself! And I determined at that point never to rule out one-half of the human race in advance as potential partners. I've been married. I'm intercontinental, not bicoastal.

I'm not going to talk much more about the old days because I don't like talking about the good old days. I don't think those were the good old days in AA; I think *these* are the good old days. AA is at least 205 reasons better today than it was in 1945 and all 205 of you are sitting right there. Look around; look at yourselves. You're beautiful! We are *far* better off now than we were then, far better off.

We did the best we could with what we had, and I was lucky enough to fall into the hands of two homosexual persons in AA, one man and one woman. And in those days, we were not closeted. In 1945, we were sealed in vaults! But we had that x-ray vision; we spotted each other and, dear God, bless their hearts, one of them is still alive. One is gone, but we remained friends all her life, and all his life; he is still living. We've remained friends all this time. And we held hands desperately together, very much, because we were the only three we saw staying sober. We'd see people coming in who were gay, obviously, and then they would leave. Only three of us seemed to be staying sober and that was very frightening, very frightening indeed.

The Third Tradition was not written when I arrived in AA in 1945. The Traditions were not to be written until Bill started a series of articles in the *Grapevine* in 1946 called "Twelve Points to Assure AA's Future," and the Third Tradition was one of them.

By the way, someone asked me a few weeks ago if I had actually met Bill Wilson. I stopped to think about it, and I said, "No, I never did"; nobody did. Bill was just there. We didn't make historic records; we didn't know we were doing anything historic! It's a wonder we have any history at all because we were too busy trying to stay sober. You know, to find a place to live, and get jobs, and get straightened out sexually and domestically, or to stay out of jail, running away from process servers—we had a lot of problems and we had to stay sober on top of all that. So you didn't "meet Bill." Nobody introduced you to him. Bill was just there all the time, and he was having his problems, too.

One of his big problems was we were jumping all over him all the time. As you know, years later he said that in writing the Big Book, he eventually became not the author but the referee. He would write a chapter and read it aloud to the members in New York, he'd send it out to Akron and they would read it out there, and then everybody would jump all over the little chapter and mail it back to him, and he would have to write it all over again.

And now he was trying out these Traditions on us. Beginning in 1946, and every Sunday afternoon, as many of us as could would go to his home in Bedford Falls, New York—Stepping Stones, where Lois lives now—and Bill would read to us what he'd written about the Traditions, and we would all tell him what was wrong with it and stomp all over it and he'd mail it to Akron, and they'd do the same thing. He had to be the referee.

I'm going to read you a few lines from the book *Twelve Steps and Twelve Traditions,* in the section on Tradition Three. I want you to hear it as it was written here and [then] hear it in another way, in Bill's voice, and you will hear a difference. And when you read it the next time, it will have a special meaning for all of us.

Bill wrote:

> On the AA calendar, it was Year Two. In that time, nothing could be seen but two struggling, nameless groups of alcoholics trying to hold their faces up to the light.
> A newcomer appeared at one of these groups, knocked on the door and asked to be let in. He talked frankly with that group's oldest member. He soon proved that his was a desperate case,

and that above all he wanted to get well. "But," he asked, "will you let me join your group? Since I am the victim of another addiction even worse stigmatized than alcoholism, you may not want me among you. Or will you?"

[Barry continues] "There was the dilemma," Bill wrote. "What should the group do?" This was published in 1952.

In 1968, the last time he was able to address the General Service Conference before he died, Bill made a talk on all the Traditions. I was there because it was my job to write the conference report; I wrote the conference reports for many years. Listening to Bill give his talk on the Traditions was old hat, I'd heard it many times and I didn't pay attention; but recently a dear friend of ours in Brooklyn called me and said, "I have found something quite remarkable that Bill said in 1968, and you should hear this tape."

The General Service Conference, for those of you who don't know, consists of a group of people elected from all the states and all the Canadian provinces. We get together once a year and spend a week fighting and arguing and talking—just as we do [at our regular AA meetings]. They have no power whatsoever. They could go there and pass all kinds of laws and we would pay no attention to them. *[Laughter]* Drunks don't take orders; you know that!

On the opening night of the General Service convention in 1968, where there were lots of non-AA guests, Bill made a talk on all the Traditions; and here's what he said this time when he gave the talk. I'm going to play the tape for you. He had emphysema very badly so it was not easy for him to talk, but I think you will hear it.

[The audience is silent while Barry adjusts the portable cassette player he has brought with him to the podium. After a moment, Bill Wilson's voice enters the auditorium over the sound system, accompanied by intermittent static and the soft hiss of the old recording. He speaks slowly, and although his breathing is labored, his voice is commanding and clear.]

At about year two of the Akron Group, a poor devil came to Dr. Bob in a grievous state, he could qualify as an alcoholic alright. And he said, "Dr. Bob, I've got a real problem to pose to you. I don't know if I could join AA, because I'm a sex deviate."

Well, that had to go out to the group conscience. You know, up 'till then it was supposed that any society could say who was going to join it. And pretty soon, the group conscience began to seethe and boil, and it boiled over.

"Under no circumstances could we have such a pall, such a disgrace, among us!" said a great many. And you know right then, our destiny hung on a razor's edge over this single case. In other words, would there be rules that could exclude so-called "undesirables?"

And that caused us in that time, and for quite a time, respecting this single case, to ponder, "What is more important—the reputation that we shall have, what people shall think? Or is it our character? And who are we, considering our records? Alcoholism is quite as unlovely. Who are we to deny a man his opportunity? Any man or woman."

And finally, the day of resolution came. A bunch of us were sitting in Dr. Bob's living room, arguing, "What to do?" Whereupon dear old Bob looked around, and blandly said, "Isn't it time folks, to ask ourselves, 'What would the Master do in a situation like this?' Would he turn this man away?"

And that was the beginning of the AA Tradition that any man who has a drinking problem is a member of AA if he says so, not whether we say so.

Now, I think the import of this on the common welfare has already been staggering, because it takes in even more territory than the confines of our fellowship; it takes in the whole world of alcoholics. Their charter to freedom to join AA is assured...

[Barry stops the tape.] So there it is in his words. *[The audience sits silently for a minute, stunned, and then gives a tremendous round of applause.]*[3]

I'm glad, however, that when Bill wrote the chapter, he opened the door even wider by not pinning it down to any one addiction or any one condition. The man said he had an addiction even more stigmatized than alcoholism, and that could be anything! And so it opened the door for millions and millions of people to come into AA, who otherwise thought they could not come into AA.

I have to go back now just a minute and tell you about a couple of experiences I had in my first year. I had this woman member and two other good women members who were friends of Bill's, older women. They had no doubt that I was a gay man and I didn't mind them knowing—they had lived in Paris much of their lives. One of these three women, by the way, was a lesbian, but this was never announced. She was always in the closet except to her very closest friends. Bill knew, of course.[4]

"Barry, we keep seeing fellows turn up here and not stay sober and it has been suggested that maybe there should be special meetings for gay people. What do you think of that?"

I thought, *Well, I don't know.* I wasn't sure I could handle that many gay people in an AA meeting! *[Laughter]* You know, I was still in my closet, my vault!

They said, "Let's talk to Bill about it," and a luncheon date was set up. The three ladies and I went to have lunch with Bill. They told Bill this story. I didn't speak up.

"Bill, we keep seeing homosexual men turn up in AA and they don't seem to stay around; they leave. Do you think it might be a good idea for these fellows to have their own meeting? . . ."

And Bill said, "Well, you know, it might be the best thing that ever came down the pike in AA. I don't know. I tell you, let's think about it. Now, Barry, can you stay sober a little while longer? How long have you been sober?"

I told him I'd been sober almost a year.

"Well, you've got friends, you could talk to these people, obviously, and you can talk to me. So do you think you could maybe make it for eighteen months? Stay sober a little while longer before we get into this?"

"Oh, yes, I think I can."

"Alright," he said, "After you've been sober about eighteen months or two years, come back and we'll talk it over." Well, of course, by the time two years had passed, the place was *alive* with AA members, homosexual, bisexual, and everything else, and transvestites, and it didn't matter to anybody. All over New York, there was this kind of member.

Now, I know from hearing a man in New Orleans that there was another city in which a group did try to set up a gay meeting early in AA history. This was in 1947, again, before the Traditions were written. Bill was in Boston making a speech trying to sell those damned Traditions of his and people were very bored. *[Laughter]* After he got through talking—Bill always knew when he was boring and if you went up afterward and said, "That was a good talk, Bill," he'd say, "Don't ever tell me that, you know I bored the pants off them; it was awful!"

So these three fellows in Boston came up to him after his talk. They said, "We have a very special problem we want to talk to you about." Bill knew what the problem was like that *[Barry snaps his fingers]*.

Bill says, "Wait a minute. Before you tell me what the problem is, are you willing to go to any lengths to stay sober?"

They said, "Yes!"

"Well, what is your problem?"

"We want to set up a meeting for gay men."

And Bill said, "Well, if that's the lengths you must go to, then go do it. Why not? Go do it!"

I'm sorry to report that the group didn't last very long. The only place they could find to meet was the basement of the YMCA and it just didn't work. *[The audience chuckles; Barry gives a little cough.]*[5]

I don't know how I stayed sober that first year; really, I don't think I tried to change. I memorized the Steps in case someone asked me, you know, for a spot check. I memorized them but I did nothing about them, but I did the things they told me to do, which would keep me dry. I didn't take the first drink, which seemed very sensible, and I did my turn sitting at the desk of the old clubhouse. We didn't have an office; we had an old clubhouse in Manhattan. It's no longer there, but as long as it stood there, I went back once a year to look at it. It was a marvelous old building, an old abandoned church.

One day I was doing my turn at the desk, answering telephones and greeting the people who walked in, and there came in, sent by a policeman on the corner, a black man. We had at that time no black AA members. We had seen a few black people come into the meetings and had tried very hard to befriend them and talk to them, but they did not stay with us. I think they found that, as they put it so beautifully, "It was too damned white." It wasn't for them and they left.

This man who was black walked in and he said, "The policeman on the corner told me that maybe you could help me." He was not only black but he had long blond hair, like Veronica Lake. *[Laughter and applause]* He was a real artist with makeup. He was beautifully made up, and strapped to his back he had his entire worldly belongings.

"I just came out of prison," he said, "I'm a dope fiend," a phrase then in use, "and I am also an alcoholic, and I need help desperately."

Well, I was the last person in the world to know what to do. I ran around trying to get someone in the office to come help me, and many found they had to play poker that afternoon. They didn't want to help. They wouldn't touch this with a ten-foot pole! Except one woman, one marvelous old woman came and sat there for long time and talked to him. But we didn't know where to start. How do you start helping somebody like this who had so many problems?

None of those people could give me the answer, so I said, "I'm going to call the person I know has been sober the longest," and I called Bill.

"Bill, here's the problem. This man is here . . ." I told him exactly what the man looked like and what he'd told us. "I got someone to take the poor guy out and get him a cup of coffee to start with. What should we do? He needs all kinds of help."

Bill was quiet a minute, then he said, "Well, now, did you say he is a drunk?"

"Oh, yes," I said, "we can all tell that—" *[Laughter]* "Right off the bat we could tell that!"

And Bill said, "I think that is the only question we have any right to ask. It is up to us now to help him." *[There is thunderous applause and cheering.]*

I'm sorry to say I don't know what happened to the man; he disappeared. Somebody else came on duty and I left. I don't know what ever happened to him; we never saw him again. I hope he made it somewhere, someplace, sometime.

The next thing that happened to me in my particular history with gay people and the Third Tradition came in 1973 and 1974 with some people from Southern California; God bless them. A lot of marvelous things happen in Southern California.[6] These fellows from California started telephoning New York and writing to New York, saying, "We want to be listed in the AA world directory as a gay group."

Ah. Problem! The General Service Office staff has no power to do anything except what they are authorized to do by the General Service Conference, which meets once a year. The staff took the subject to the conference and said, "You'll have to tell us what you want us to do, whether you want us to list these groups or not."

And when we start talking about listing a group as a gay group or a lesbian group, we are getting into some areas that are not terribly black and white. We are beginning to tread kind of closely to several Traditions. What about the tradition of inclusiveness? If you set up gay groups, would they exclude other people?

That was one of the big arguments against it at the conference in 1973, and the discussion got going hot and heavy; it was really very distressing. Finally, at the end of the afternoon discussion, which was so hot and heavy, the chairman had a very smart idea—a very smart AA idea: he tabled the matter until next year. *[Laughter]*

This meant it was on the conference agenda for the next year and when the conference met in 1974 and it came time to discuss this question, three of the delegates—one from Southern California, one from Chicago, and one from Washington DC—had done their homework. They'd been to all the gay groups they could find and they had talked to every gay member they could find. These men had talked to their constituencies, you might say, so they knew what they were talking about. "They are very good AA," they said. "If they want to be listed as gay, let them be listed as gay. Why not?" One of them reported that we probably wouldn't even have enough people to man our volunteer desks if it weren't for the gay people. But that was not enough to settle the argument.

The argument went on into the evening and finally the discussion was called off because everything was getting pretty steamed. The next evening's agenda was wiped off and devoted to this question. It had to be settled. Now, it is the policy of the conference almost never to settle any issue without almost total unanimity—we don't want to settle any matter simply by majority vote since it would leave an unhappy minority. You want almost total unanimity at the General Service Conference.

I'm sitting there taking the notes and listening to this debate. I'm hearing some people say, "Oh my god, are we going to let the queers in?" And, "If we list queers, what are you going to do next year, list rapists? Are you going to have rapists' groups?" And then somebody else said, "Yeah, and then child molesters?" Well, if you have read any of the literature on child molestation, raping, and wife beating, you know there's a little alcoholism involved; so I'm pretty certain there are wife beaters, child molesters, and rapists in AA, aren't you? And they deserve our love.

One man gave a speech about these deviates, as he called them, as Bill used the old phrase "sex deviate." The delegate from one of the northern states or Canadian provinces that year was a tiny woman, and when he made some remark about sex deviates, she ran to the microphone. She pulled the microphone down to her face—she was only about three feet tall—and in a high, squeaky little voice she said, "Where I come from, *alcoholics* are considered deviates." *[There is a thunderous burst of applause. When it has subsided, Barry continues.]*

About that time, a nonalcoholic doctor on our board of trustees— our board of trustees has twenty-one people; fourteen are AA members and seven are not. They're just our front men. *[Laughter]* One of them was the treasurer; as a custom we always make sure that the treasurer is a nonalcoholic, for pretty obvious reasons. This nonalcoholic doctor, whom I had known long before he got onto our board, came up to my little niche where I was sitting in the back taking notes.

"Barry, when you first listed women's groups did they go through all this?"

"No . . ."

"Well, when you first listed young people's groups in the directory, did you go through all this?"

And I said, "No, we didn't do this."

He walked over to the microphone, and I'm not going to tell you his name, but I think we owe this man a great debt of love. He walked to the microphone and said, "I understand that when you listed young people's groups, you did not go through these shenanigans. Is that right?"

And everybody said, "Yes . . ."

"And that when you listed women's groups you didn't go through all this folderol did you?"

And everybody said, "No, we didn't do it then."

"Well, what in the world are you picking on *these* guys for?" and he took his seat.

And you could feel the room tangibly change at that moment. And the chairman of the conference at that minute also felt the change, and he called the question. And out of 131 votes that year, 128 of the people voting said we should list gay groups if they wished to be so listed. Only two people voted against it, which was very, very thrilling. *[Applause]*

And then to put the icing on the cake, immediately after the vote was announced, somebody said, "I want to propose a resolution. That it is the consensus of the conference that no AA group, anywhere, of any kind, should ever turn a newcomer away from his or her first meeting," and that was passed unanimously.

That was a great moment in our AA history, when we really began to apply the Third Tradition. Some of us were already, of course, preparing for things like this to happen, looking down the road apiece.

One of the AA books I wrote, which I wrote in 1972, is called *Living Sober*. You don't have to read it, but if you want to read it sometime, if you read between the lines, you'll find several things that hold meanings for us that aren't obvious to other people. I think they took out one line as a little bit too campy, something about "cruising along—" *[laughter]* "searching for love in all the wrong places" *[more laughter]*. I think they took it out because somebody didn't understand it. Writing for AA is fun; you have so many editors.

But in 1976, again the pressure had risen from around the country that we must have a pamphlet for gay people. There was also pressure on us that we must have a pamphlet put out for Native Americans, that we should have a pamphlet for Hispanics, that we should publish a pamphlet for black people, that we should publish one for young people, that we should publish one for older people, and I'll never forget one delegate on the Literature Committee that year who said, "I think we should also publish a pamphlet for illiterates." I looked at the chairman, the chairman looked at me, and we both looked at the secretary. This man meant it! I don't know in what language he thought . . .[7]

They decided to try and respond to these pressures by putting out a pamphlet entitled *So You Think You Are Different*. I didn't like that title. I objected to it, and started whining about it—which I learned in my first year was a very good manipulative trick; just keep whining long enough and someone will find a way around your whine, or get rid of you—and I kept whining because I thought it sounded snide! "So, you think you're different, huh?" And finally someone said, "What do you think of the title *Do You Think You're Different?*" Ah, that doesn't sound snide at all! They said, "We will have to hire a writer to write this pamphlet," and I said, "I have all the stories ready." *[Laughter]*

There it is *[holding up a copy of* Do You Think You're Different?*]*; you've read it, maybe. We were ready for this one: "Do you think you're different." And it does have black stories, and Indian stories, old people stories, young people stories, all kinds of stories, and a number of stories in here by people who are gay but never talk about being gay, but talk about other aspects about being different, which I think is marvelous.

I believe that the Third Tradition is a great blessing for us. It has given us a double whammy of love when we get together at Round-ups like this. You know, the other people don't get to have these love feasts like we do. However, I realize, as this goes on, that there grows for us some extra responsibility. I am also impressed, and a little bit ashamed, by the fact that we haven't yet learned to love enough. I think if the Third Tradition means anything, it means that I owe un-conditional love to the next drunk that walks in the door, even if that drunk happens to be a former Miss America, or a well-known TV evangelist, or a California legislator.[8] I have a lot of learning about love to do. But I think we have to do it.

I happen to have in my keeping at home the original manuscript of the Big Book, the typescript as it went to the printer. My will says it belongs to the fellowship but it is in my keeping until I die, then it goes to the archives. You can get copies of this from the General Service Office in New York.

By the way, if you've not seen it in typescript, the printer's manu-script is the one to look at. I tell you, it's a gas! Do you want to hear "How It Works" in the Big Book as it was originally written? When it gets down to the point where it says, ". . . that God could and would if sought," the original manuscript says, ". . . and you must find him now." *[Laughter]* "If not, go out and drink some more, then read the book again." *[More laughter]* "And if you still don't find him, throw the book away." *[The audience howls.]* They had an awful problem editing that manuscript, as you can see![9]

I found written in the flyleaf of the manuscript, some handwriting done in pencil, and I recognized the words instantly. I thought, *I wonder why it's written in pencil in the flyleaf and not typed in typescript?* And I got hold of our archivist Nell, who was Bill's secretary for many years, and we began to run this down.

Nell recognized the handwriting as that of a man named Hank, who was more of a promoter than Bill was—and that was a lot of promoting. Hank was pushing the manuscript very hard, pushing the book, and pushing Bill to get it finished, and [one night] he heard Bill telling his story again, what Bill called "the bedtime story."

Bill had a marvelous way of talking about his experiences. He called his spiritual awakening that he had in Town's hospital—where he said he'd had "the wind of the great spirit" blowing through him and all this—he called that his "hot flash."

Telling his story, Bill told about a morning when he was living in Brooklyn Heights with Lois. The house is still there. Brooklyn [AA] has put out a little pamphlet for the AA fiftieth anniversary *[holding up a copy of the pamphlet]*; there's the house and there's the kitchen underneath the stoop. Although he'd been a Wall Street hotshot, Bill was unable to work because of his drinking and Lois was supporting the two of them by working in a department store. Bill was sitting there one morning with a bottle of gin, bathtub gin in 1934, when he got a telephone call from an old drinking chum named Ebby.

He hadn't seen Ebby in years, and he loved to drink with Ebby. He and Ebby had done some marvelous things together, some really ridiculous wild things. Once upon a time, Ebby and Bill drove off a highway right into a kitchen. The lady in the kitchen was a bit disturbed *[laughter]* but Ebby said, "Don't be alarmed. Could you spare a cup of coffee?" Bill and Ebby had some wild escapades together.

When Ebby came over, he walked in sober. Bill had never seen Ebby sober and—of course, he was as drunk on pity at that moment as he was on gin—Bill pushed a water glass full of gin across the table to Ebby and said, "Have a drink."

Ebby said, "Nope, I've got religion."

Bill's heart sank. He thought Ebby was much too bright for that. He said, "Oh my god, what brand did you get?" We talked in terms of brands, in many of our drinking days. Ebby said, "I don't know if you could call it any brand. I just ran into this bunch of fellows and we have six little ideas. And we simply do these things and I don't seem to want to drink anymore." The Brooklyn pamphlet has these six little ideas that later turned into the Twelve Steps.

Bill was quite taken, when he heard these six ideas. He knew his own case was hopeless; he and Lois had already been told by Dr. Silkworth that his case was hopeless and that if he ever drank again, he would wind up either with brain damage in a hospital as a vegetable for the rest of his life, or in a drunkard's grave very soon; so Bill knew there was no hope for him. And he certainly was not about to be religious.

So when Bill told this part of the story [again] about Ebby, Hank was sitting there and he realized that it was not in the typescript, that it had been left out. Like a lot of us, this almost didn't get in. It was not connected anywhere. And thank God, Hank wrote it in pencil on the flyleaf and told the printer, "Put this in on page twelve."

I know that this is on page twelve because I kept searching for these familiar lines in the typescript but couldn't find them. Now of course I know what happened: Hank simply gave them to the printer. And this is exactly what they say. *[He pauses.]* It's hard to read because I choke up. It's also hard to read because Hank was writing fast [as Bill relayed the story], and used abbreviations. He wrote:

Despite the living example of my friend, there remained in me the vestiges of my old prejudice. The word God still aroused a certain antipathy. When the thought was expressed that there might be a God personal to me this feeling was intensified. I didn't like the idea. I could go for such concepts as Creative Intelligence, Universal Mind, or Spirit of Nature, but I resisted the thought of a Czar of the Heavens, however loving His sway might be. I have since talked with scores of men who felt the same way. My friend suggested what then seemed a novel idea.

You'll find this next idea in italics; it's underscored in Hank's handwriting:

He said, *"Why don't you choose your own conception of God?"*
That statement hit me hard. It melted the icy intellectual mountains in whose shadows I had lived and shivered many years. I stood in the sunlight at last. *It was only a matter of being*

willing to believe in a Power greater than myself. Nothing more was required of me to make my beginning. I saw that growth could start from that point. Upon a foundation of complete willingness, I might build what I saw in my friend. Would I have it? Of course I would!

It seems to me that when Ebby said to Bill, "Why don't you choose your own conception of God," that he laid the foundation down for the Third Tradition. Surely if we are not to impose our own conceptions of God on anybody else, and we don't want anyone imposing theirs on us, surely none of us has any business imposing our sexual codes on other people. And we don't want them to impose theirs on us.

When I was drunk I often used to say, "Why me?" Why was I the one picked out for all this suffering? Even after I got sober that went on for a long time, "Why me? Why can so many people drink and get by with it? Why me?" I had that feeling again a few years ago when my lover died, after twenty-six years. "Why me? Why does it happen to me?"

I've since come to learn, since come to understand, since come to believe, why *not* me? Why not me? And some days, some evenings, out of the corner of my eye, I think I get just a slight glimpse of a running-away shadow, and that's the reason why it's me.

I think all my life I've been on my way to be here, at home, with you tonight. Thank you.

[The audience leaps to their feet, cheering.]

Chapter 3

Alcoholism and Homosexuality: A Brief History of Treatment

> You're right about your homosexual activities being directly triggered by your drinking. I'd go so far to say now it's possible you'd stop all of it if you were sober.
>
> Dr. Lawrence Hatterer
> *Changing Homosexuality in the Male*

Introduction

From the late 1800s until the 1970s in the United States, most physicians, psychiatrists, psychologists, and other medical scientists believed that alcoholism and homosexuality were etiologically—that is, causally—linked. In the early 1900s, Dr. Sigmund Freud introduced the idea that a whole host of conditions, including alcoholism and homosexuality, were the result of an underlying psychological pathology or illness. According to Dr. Freud and his many followers, in inebriates, homosexuals, and patients with many other types of conditions, the root of this illness could be traced to immature or maladapted sexual development.

In *Slaying the Dragon: The History of Addiction Treatment and Recovery in America,* historian William White writes:

> The evolving psychoanalytic literature linked substance abuse to a wide variety of maladies: "arrested psycho-sexual development," "impulse neurosis," "character disorders," "perversions,"

The History of Gay People in Alcoholics Anonymous
Published by The Haworth Press, Inc., 2007. All rights reserved.
doi:10.1300/5699_03

"oral-narcissistic fixations resulting from forced weaning," "primary maternal identification," "compulsion neurosis," "masochism," "slow suicide," "infantile narcissism," "mother fixation," "fear of castration," and "latent homosexuality." (White 1998, p. 96)

White found the first psychoanalytic interpretation of habitual drunkenness in an article by Karl Abraham titled, "The Psychological Relations Between Sexuality and Alcoholism," published in the *International Journal of Psycho-Analysis* in 1908:

> Abraham attributed chronic drunkenness in men to an unresolved oral dependency that resulted in alcohol's replacement of women as a sexual object. According to Abraham, drinking was the sexual activity of the alcoholic. He proclaimed that "every drinking bout is tinged with homosexuality" and that men grasp at alcohol as a substitute for their "vanishing procreative power." This view of alcoholism as a manifestation of latent homosexuality continued well into the second half of the 20th century." (Ibid., p. 96)

While homosexuality underpinned alcoholism, drinking was seen to cause homosexual acts. In other words, homosexuals' alcoholism was caused by their homosexuality, and their homosexuality was caused by their excessive drinking.

In the 1950s and 1960s, a physician named Dr. Lawrence Hatterer treated over 600 men for homosexuality at the Payne Whitney Psychiatric Institute and the Cornell University Medical Center in New York. According to a recent review of Hatterer's book *Changing Homosexuality in the Male,* published in 1970, the first step in treatment was to get patients to identify the triggers that stimulated and perpetuated their homosexuality, including personal associations (friends, lovers, and other gay people); homosexual behavior, such as going to bars and cruising places; and the use of drugs and alcohol (Phillips 2004).

Despite the fact that no direct connection has ever been established between them, the association between homosexuality and alcoholism continues to persist. Here is a recent example from the June 16, 1998, issue of the *New York Times:*

In an interview about his personal beliefs, Senator Trent Lott, the majority leader, told a conservative talk show host today that homosexuality is a sin and then compared it to such personal problems as alcoholism, kleptomania, and "sex addiction. . . . You still love that person and you should not try to mistreat them or treat them as outcasts." (Mitchell 1998, p. A24)

Treatments for Alcoholism

White describes in detail the methods used to treat alcoholism in the early part of the twentieth century. These included special diets, exercise regimens, constructive leisure, constructive work (for example, tending crops or livestock on a farm or performing maintenance at a hospital facility), and exposing the patient to natural elements in the form of "cures." These included gold cures, steel cures, iron cures, sun cures, air cures, and bark cures. Water cures, one of the most frequently employed, included hot baths, cold baths, steam baths, sponge baths, enemas, douches, hot water packs, cold water packs, and drinking large quantities of water.

Drug-based therapies for alcoholism in this period included administering morphine, chloral hydrate, and/or paraldehyde (a sedative used to treat convulsive disorders), along with mixtures called "tonics" that included, along with the previous drugs, strychnine, atropine, capsicum (hot pepper), passiflora, hydrastis, gentian, cinchona, hyoscine, and scopolamine. Psychological treatment for alcoholism involved psychoanalysis and other types of psychotherapy aimed at bringing unconscious desires and motivations to the patient's conscious level, the theory being that once the patient was conscious of these he or she would be freed of the compulsion to drink.

Surgical treatments were also used. White provides this account of the first lobotomy performed on an alcoholic in the United States by two physicians:

The first psychosurgery procedures in the United States were conducted by Drs. Walter Freeman and James Watts in 1936. Their fifteenth lobotomy patient was an alcoholic who had been subjected to this procedure on the grounds that the surgical alteration of personality would alter the patient's pathological craving for alcohol. Following this procedure, the patient dressed and, pulling a hat down over his bandaged head, slipped out of the hospital in search of a drink. Freeman and Watts spent Christmas Eve, 1936, searching the bars for this patient, whom they eventually found and returned to the hospital in a state of extreme intoxication. (White 1998, p. 94)

White concludes his remarks on lobotomy with these disturbing statistics:

Between 1944 and 1960, 100,000 psychosurgery procedures [lobotomies] were performed in the U.S. The number of alcoholics and addicts who underwent this procedure is unknown, but the literature on psychosurgery noted the viability of this technique in treating "compulsive hedonias": alcoholism, drug addiction, excessive eating, and sexual deviations. (Ibid., p. 95)

Treatments for Homosexuality

Many of the techniques used to treat alcoholism were also used to cure homosexuality, not surprisingly, with similar results. In *Gay American History: Lesbians and Gay Men in the U.S.A.,* historian Jonathan Katz documents treatments for homosexuality in the United States during this same period, 1900 to 1970. In a chilling presentation of the material, Katz quotes directly from journal articles written by the doctors developing and administering these treatments. When *Gay American History* was first published in 1976, many of the treatments he described were still in use.[1]

In his introduction to the chapter titled "Treatment: 1884-1974," Katz writes:

The treatment of [l]esbians and [g]ay men by psychiatrists and psychologists constitutes one of the more lethal forms of homosexual oppression. Among the treatments are surgical measures: castration, hysterectomy, and vasectomy. In the 1800s, surgical removal of the ovaries and of the clitoris is discussed as a "cure" for various forms of female "erotomania," including, it seems, [l]esbianism. Lobotomy was performed as late as 1951. A variety of drug therapies have been employed, including the administration of hormones, LSD, sexual stimulants, and sexual depressants. Hypnosis, used on [g]ay people in America as early as 1899, was still being used to treat such "deviant behavior" in 1967. Other documented "cures" are shock treatment, both electric and chemical; aversion therapy, employing nausea-inducing drugs, electric shock, and/or negative verbal suggestion; and a type of behavior therapy called "sensitization," intended to increase heterosexual arousal, making ingenious use of pornographic photos. Often homosexuals have been the subjects of Freudian psychoanalysis and other varieties of individual and group psychotherapy. Some practitioners (a Catholic one is quoted) have treated homosexuals by urging an effort of the will directed toward the goal of sexual abstinence. Primal therapists, vegetotherapists, and the leaders of each new psychological fad have had their say about treating homosexuals. (Katz 1976, pp. 197-198)

An Alcoholics Anonymous (AA) member named George D. shared his experience at a workshop at the 1980 International AA Convention in New Orleans:

My family doctor [sent] me to a psychiatrist he thought might help me. . . . I went to see the psychiatrist; he gave me truth serum and couldn't get a word out of me—I could not talk about the most important thing I needed to, to get well. Finally, I mentioned to him some of the things about my homosexual feelings. He never said a word to me about it. He said, "You are very very depressed, and we are going to have to give you shock treatment." Of course, I was depressed! I was drinking alcohol, which is one of the worst depressants you can take. And he had me on a medication that I discovered was also a depressant.

I took six of those things. . . . It was like having someone run electricity behind your eyes from this side to this side. You feel yourself convulsing, and then they hold you down, and you're gone. But some of this had to do with my underlying feeling that I wanted to be well.

I didn't know where I was, and nobody was giving me the right information. I discovered, really not so long ago, through another therapist, that the reason he gave me the shock treatment was to cure my homosexuality. That was the one way I would no longer be an alcoholic and I would no longer be depressed. I am happy to report that I am still a homosexual.

Because that doctor wasn't making any progress with me he did finally say, "Maybe you might go to AA. You might learn something from them." I was willing to try anything, so I went to AA. What a wonderful bunch of people!

I stopped drinking. But there were those feelings inside of me that I couldn't talk to anyone about. I'd been sober a little while and was speaking at a meeting in the Bronx. A man at that meeting who had obviously been drinking raised his hand to talk and a guy in the back of the room yelled out, "You can't help him! He'll never get sober, he's a homosexual!"

I sort of hurt inside, and I felt very frightened, but I also have a certain amount of gall, and I told the man who raised his hand, "If you wait for me, I'll talk to you after the meeting."

I don't know what happened to him, but that was the starting point for me. I began to look at myself and wonder, *Was it true that I could never got sober because I was a homosexual?*

Eugenics

Due to the work of gay historians like Katz, we know today that sexual surgery was considered a viable option for treatment of homosexuality in the first half of the twentieth century. But very few people are aware that thousands of alcoholics were routinely subjected to sexual surgery during the same period. The surgery was not to cure their alcoholism (though this was sometimes listed as a positive side effect), but to prevent them from passing their genes on to future generations. Starting in the late 1920s, alcoholics—along with many other people categorized as "genetically defective," including "sex deviates"—were targeted by a group of scientists who believed that human beings could be systematically improved through "better breeding," a science they called eugenics. Proponents of eugenics maintained that society's problems were the result of "cumulative hereditary degeneracy"; that is, inferior genetic characteristics were passed on in increasingly severe forms to successive generations. Eugenicists mounted a national campaign to encourage people with "good genetic characteristics" to marry and procreate. People with "bad genetic characteristics" were discouraged, and ultimately prevented from doing so.[2]

> There is no longer any questioning of the fact that the degenerate class is increasing out of all proportion to the increase of the general population. . . . [This class of degenerates includes] most of the insane, the epileptic, the imbecile, the idiotic, the sexual perverts; many of the confirmed inebriates, prostitutes, tramps and criminals as well as the habitual paupers found in our county poor asylums; also many of the children in our orphan homes . . .

> Dr. H. C. Sharpe, physician at the Indiana Reformatory
> "The Sterilization of Degenerates" (1909)
> Paper presented to the American Prison Association

Eugenics achieved widespread acceptance in the United States and Europe in the 1930s and 1940s. It formed the basis of U.S. immigration policy, and the laws that regulated who was allowed to marry whom. State antimiscegenation laws prohibited individuals from different "races" from marrying. Racial characteristics included skin and hair color, as well as other "genetically determined" characteristics, including blindness, deafness, alcoholism, "insanity," and "feeble-mindedness." In *The Surgical Solution: A History of Involuntary Sterilization in the United States,* Philip Reilly (1991) documents the history of Eugenics in America. Between 1905 and 1922, thirty bills permitting the sterilization of institutionalized persons were passed in eighteen states.

> The Iowa law gave the state board of parole the power to sterilize those persons who "would produce children with tendency to disease, deformity, crime, insanity, feeble-mindedness, idiocy, imbecility, epilepsy, or alcoholism, or if the physical or mental condition of any such inmate will probably be materially improved thereby, or if such inmate is an epileptic or syphilitic, or gives evidence, while an inmate of such institution, that he or she is a moral or sexual pervert. (Reilly 1991, p. 53)

Between 1907 and 1963, over 60,000 Americans were involuntarily sterilized through state-conducted programs that targeted institutionalized people (Ibid., p. 94). It is not known how many were sterilized because of alcoholism, though in his brief treatment of the topic, William White observes that Reilly's figure (60,000) does not include anyone "deinstitutionalized contingent upon sterilization." White writes:

> While sterilization of alcoholics was "voluntary" in many states, by mid-century there existed a coercive influence that could be brought to bear on such individuals. In the 1960s, this author interviewed a number of alcoholic women who had been committed to state psychiatric facilities in the 1940s and 1950s. Many of these women reported that they were not discharged until they submitted to "voluntary" sterilization. In reviewing the medical records of these women, it became apparent that they were subjected to pressure for sterilization the moment that excessive drinking appeared in their history. (White 1998, p. 89)

As corrosive and damaging as eugenics was in the United States, its most dramatic implementation occurred in Nazi Germany, where it formed the basis of the Third Reich's racial purity laws.

Persecution of Homosexuals and Alcoholics
in Nazi Germany

Most people today know that homosexuals were among those persecuted in Nazi Germany. Between 1933 and 1945, under Paragraph 175 of the German Penal Code, an estimated 100,000 men were arrested for homosexuality in Germany. Of these, 50,000 were sent to prison and 15,000 were sent to concentration camps (Epstein and Friedman 2000). But few are aware that alcoholics were also targeted by the Third Reich, under Germany's eugenics-based medical and "social compatibility" laws.

Along with thousands of other "genetically defective" people—the blind, deaf, epileptic, disabled, and mentally ill—alcoholics were routinely interred, sterilized, and, later, killed in Germany's concentration camps. These were the people on whom the Nazis first developed and refined the mechanisms used later in the camps to exterminate millions. The process began with sterilization and ended with the gas chambers.

In "Alcohol and the State in Nazi Germany, 1933-1945," published in 1991 in *Drinking: Behavior and Belief in Modern History,* Hermann Fahrenkrug shows that, between 1933 and 1945 in Germany, under the Law for the Prevention of Descendents Affected by Hereditary Disorders, an estimated 20,000 to 30,000 alcoholics were sterilized. This was a mere fraction, he notes, of the 150,000 to 200,000 alcoholics marked for sterilization by German racial hygiene specialists and the Nazi health management.

In 1935, the Third Reich's Marriage Health Law forbade marriage "if one member of the engaged pair suffers from a mental disturbance," including "those with alcoholism of every form and cause" (Fahrenkrug 1991).

It was eugenicists in the United States who first developed the codes and symbols used to classify people they saw as a threat to a healthy society. These were adopted and later expanded upon by the Nazis. In Germany Jews were made to wear yellow stars and homosexuals to wear pink triangles. People sent to the concentration camps for being "asocial" or "antisocial"—in other words, "deemed hostile to the existence of society, or the principles on which it is founded"—were made to wear a black triangle. In addition to alcoholics, this category included vagrants, prostitutes, thieves, gypsies, and lesbians (Edelheit and Edelheit 1994).

Under wartime conditions in Germany (1939 to 1945), Fahrenkrug concludes:

> [Alcoholics] already marginalized during peacetime as hereditary inferiors, psychopaths, and antisocials . . . were now declared by the leadership to be dangerous enemies of the German people. . . . The public inebriate assistance agencies concerned themselves less with cure or treatment than with security measures for the protection of the public. . . . The passage of alcohol control from the medically arranged hereditary disease law to the newly assembled "Social Inability Law" combined the existing measures of sterilization, prohibition of marriage, and security detention so as to reach a "final solution" of the alcoholic question. Socially incapable inebriates received the degrading punishment of complete exclusion from national life and were

surrendered to "annihilation through work." (Fahrenkrug 1991, pp. 330-331)

Gay people and alcoholics share a long history of being targeted and criminalized by people who claim they are a threat to society. Doctors and psychiatrists have used many of the same techniques to treat alcoholism and homosexuality, a list that would include psychotherapy, aversion therapy, drug therapy, chemical and electrical shock treatments, sterilization, lobotomy, and cold baths.

Government authorities have argued that alcoholics and homosexuals are "asocial," that is, that they are bad for society, and they have passed laws designed to circumscribe their rights in order to protect healthy and decent citizens. These laws include those designed to limit or prevent them from entering the country, from marrying, and from having children.

> Ages of experience have taught humanity that the commitment of a husband and wife to love and to serve one another promotes the welfare of children and the stability of society. Marriage cannot be severed from its cultural, religious, and natural roots without weakening the good influence of society. Government, by recognizing and protecting marriage, serves the interests of all.
>
> President George W. Bush (February 24, 2004)
> Calling for a constitutional amendment
> to deny gay Americans the right to marry

In 1967, the American Medical Association passed a resolution officially recognizing alcoholism as a disease. Six years later, in 1973, the American Psychiatric Association officially removed homosexuality from its *Diagnostic and Statistical Manual of Mental Disorders*. These acts would have profound implications for alcoholics and for gay people in the United States: for the first time in history, alcoholism was an illness and homosexuality was not.

Chapter 4

Five Views of Sober Gay Life in the 1950s and 1960s

Mr. Chairman, I realize that I am discussing a very delicate subject and I cannot lay the bones bare like I could before medical colleagues. I would like to strip the fetid, stinking flesh off of this skeleton of homosexuality and tell my colleagues of the House some of the facts of nature. I cannot expose all the putrid facts, as it would offend the sensibilities of some of you. It will be necessary to skirt some of the edges, and I use certain Latin terms to describe some of these individuals. Make no mistake, several thousand, according to police records, are now employed by the Federal Government.

> Congressman Miller (1950),
> From the floor of the House of Representatives

Ben G.

[Ben came into AA in Boston in 1952. I interviewed him at his home in San Francisco.]

I first started attending Alcoholics Anonymous (AA) meetings in Boston. Later I moved to New York. . . .

I knew people who were gay but it was a whole different world; it was a subculture. . . . At that time, I had no idea how many gay people there were. Kinsey had come out with his [report] that said 10 percent [of the population was gay], but where the heck were they?

The History of Gay People in Alcoholics Anonymous
Published by The Haworth Press, Inc., 2007. All rights reserved.
doi:10.1300/5699_04

In Boston, there were a few bars where, on a certain day, if a certain bartender was working, that a certain corner of the bar was gay. But you couldn't be sure of it. You might go there, buy a couple drinks, and find it was not a gay night, not the gay corner. But when Don VanWard was in the Napoleon Bar, it was gay in *his* corner. Oh! What a charmer he was. He played piano like a whiz and sang. People gathered around him and we had lots of fun. Then we'd go our separate ways. There was no exchanging of telephone numbers or anything. You went somewhere and did it, right then and there, or it was an ephemeral cloud that just vanished. When I got sober, this was all I had known. And I found there wasn't anything in AA either, not even an ephemeral section. . . .

At that time, I knew just one exception to the rule that anyone was welcome in AA and the exception was gay people. Read the Big Book carefully and you'll see there's never any mention of gay people. Also, as mentioned in the fifth chapter, which we read at every meeting in California, *[paraphrasing]* "There are those among us afflicted with serious mental and emotional disorders, but many of them do recover, if they are willing to be honest." And of course, I fit into that because I don't fit anywhere else. I thought, *I'm going to go through a process where they welcome everyone except me.*

I left New York in 1962 following a shattering experience. . . . The Adonis Mail Club was a way to exchange letters between gay people in different cities. They gave you the names and addresses of two gay people every month that you could write to, and they could write to me if they wanted. I have a way of archiving things, and I had carbons of all the letters I'd written and the letters I'd received and replied to.

The postal inspectors had been to see me.[1] They tried to bargain with me and told me that if I turned the files over to them, nothing would happen to me.

"Files? What do you mean, 'files'? There are no files." Of course, right behind the guy was the trunk with all the files in it!

"We can't force you," they said. "We're just trying to make it easy for you."

After they left and the door was locked, after I'd heard them down the stairs and I was sure they'd left the building, I started burning the letters. I burned them in the bathtub. I burned so many that I had to repaint. I was desperate to get the place clean. The police might have come a couple of hours after the postal inspectors. This was something McCarthy had stirred up, to "clean up the filth in the postal system."

I was called to witness against some poor man they were trying to prosecute. They sent me to Chicago and put me up in a hotel. They got awfully little from me for the money they spent. All I could say was that I'd had a letter from him. That's it. God, I felt sorry for that guy. He had an old guy who got up to defend him. Not his lawyer— this is probably one of the Mattachines. . . . He was great to do it, although I don't think it did any good.

Then the postal inspectors leveled a charge against me. I asked one of the lawyers at the Democratic Club I belonged to if he'd defend me. . . .

"Um, uh, well, I don't know," [he said].

"Please," I said. "Please! I need your help!"

Finally, he said he'd do it on one condition: "After it's over, you must never mention that I had anything to do with the case," he said. Those were the terms. We paid him $750 [$9,000 in today's currency] and he persuaded the judge to accept a plea of guilty.

"It's not in the interest of the state to have this man imprisoned," the judge said—thank God for that. . . . They put me on a year's probation.

The probation officer said, "We have to let the people closest to you know." I told him my mother already knew about it.

"I don't mean your mother. I mean your former wife."

"Wait a minute. *Former* wife," I said. "We're divorced!"

"Oh, this is a big relationship. You have children. The law says I must do it. But I can fix it so you can tell her instead of us. How would that be?"

When I met with her, she flung her arms around me and wept. "You poor man," she said.

At that point, my mother came to town. She took me out to dinner, as she often did, and asked me, "Are you free of all that?"

Remember, this was back in the hint stage. One didn't say these things. "Are you free of 'all that.'" . . . And that's where she left it. The follow-up came later.

Some people came to see me. Over the next two weeks, more people came to see me. Each time it was more painful. They convinced me that I was selfish, and wicked, and against God.

By that point, I'd got it clearly in mind that I was trying to live by the Eleventh Step, to seek, through prayer and meditation, God's will instead of my own, and I thought I was doing that.

"Well," the man said, I was not in line with "the better view" of the deity, the more "wholesome" view, and they punched another nail into me. These were Buchmanites, Moral Re-Armament people. My mother was involved in that. This was a forerunner of AA.[2]

Were you still going to meetings during this time?

Oh yes, but this never came up. I wasn't going to talk about *this* sort of thing. Wow! This would have been hot news! And you never know who is at an AA meeting. There were no safe places.

The first time I connected with other gay people in AA was in Denver [at AA's international conference in 1975]. I saw a sign in the hotel lobby that said, "Gay in AA? Meet in Room 422 at 2:00." This guy got someone to agree to let him put up the sign and about twenty of us showed up. There had been sort of a gay thing in New York when I was there. I'd asked someone about it who I knew was gay.

"We're meeting at someone's apartment," he said, "but it's full now. There's only room for nine people and we've got nine, so start [a group] of your own."

Most of us in Denver that day . . . had found somebody in AA [we'd] discovered . . . was gay, but then you don't talk about that at a meeting. So the whole thing was to try to build something we could meet at somewhere. The reaction in AA was very mixed, mostly against it. People were frightened. They thought, "We've got this much: the approval of the general public. The Lasker Award. And now *this* comes up?"[3]

The idea of Living Sober [the gay AA conference in San Francisco] was another stage in 1976, the year I came to San Francisco. We had hippies, and people who were up the ying-yang in marijuana, colorful clothes, free in the streets—all that was going on. It was terribly exciting. We had 250 people [at the first Living Sober] and it was clear that we were on the cusp of something quite new. But Living Sober wasn't an isolated event. It was part of a growing movement. San Francisco was full of that, that year. [That was the year] the California legislature repealed the statute that said being gay was a criminal offense. Once that was gone, the police no longer had a big thing to back them up. Unfortunately, the police didn't get the point as quickly as we['d] hoped.

Pucky

[Pucky grew up in an affluent family on Long Island, New York. She first began attending AA meetings in 1947 when she was twenty-two.]

I was a problem drinker. I wanted to be a writer; and a teacher who was very worried about me dragged me to an AA meeting. Many of the people [at the meeting] were students of hers, and when we arrived they all descended on us. So my plan of not saying what I was doing there went out the window. A very much older woman turned to me and said, "Is it you or your friend who has a problem?" "Oh, no, I'm the one," I said.

There was a panel of speakers that night and the older woman was on it; her name was Grace. Grace told about how she hid liquor and disguised it as medicine, which was very much my kind of thing. Another speaker talked about the alcoholic personality and the tie-up between arrogance and shyness, which I understood instantly. And that you didn't need an awful lot of willpower. In fact, they said you needed to surrender your will, which was good news to me. I'd been on all kinds of diets, and knowing sobriety wasn't going to be like going to Success School and starving was a relief—because I could keep that up [not eating] for maybe three weeks, or whatever the time period was, but not for life. I knew I didn't have any willpower.

At the end of the meeting, they said the Lord's Prayer, which made me mad. I don't know why. I'd said it all my life at every boarding school I ever went to. *I'm getting out of here,* I thought, and as I turned to leave I walked right into one of my friend's students. He was an older man, a very square fellow, and he'd had a stroke or disability that made him speak a little strangely. He asked, "Aren't you going to stay for coffee?"

I can't be rude to this man, I thought; *he's probably the only person in this city shyer than I am.* So I said I would stay.

[This man, whose name was] Bud, later became a mentor to me. He'd gone to the same college as my father and was the same kind of guy. AA was like a club, for a certain type of person. And while

I understood them, and liked them, I didn't want to become one of them. I wanted to become part of the world. That was always a very deep determination I had. . . .

I was ambitious. I wanted to be a writer, and I wanted to be a part of the world. But a person like me with two strikes against her, as far as the world was concerned, had a row to hoe to try and find out who she was, and how to pursue that without getting crucified. My stepfather was a publisher and there were writers crawling all over the house. To be a writer was not the way out of a publisher's family and I thought I'd better go in a different direction. I worked in television for forty years.

After five years in AA I had a one-night slip, because I was having some doomed romance, because I hadn't been to meetings, and because I was tied up with professional things. The next morning Bud came over and we talked. I don't remember what we talked about, but that was the end of my drinking.

I had enormous luck because I was not leveling with my AA friends about what was troubling me the most, which of course was not only the career, but the hiding, the pretending to be one thing when you are another.

What words would you have used to describe yourself then? Would you have used the word "gay"?

Then? I don't know. I was so busy *not* describing myself.

It was accepted that you didn't accept it, you ducked and lied, did what you had to do to keep away from the posse. And you really raised your eyebrows at anybody who didn't.

For the most part, I'm pretty flip. My normal communications are lighthearted, and I try to keep them that way. But I do not volunteer lies. Or say I'm one thing when I'm another. It's too much of a strain. I'm seventy-seven years old! If I weren't at peace by this time I'd be half out of my head now, wouldn't I? It's a slow, long process—not only to accept yourself, but to get really . . . annoyed at the people who wouldn't accept you. That's a lifetime proposition. Or it was for my generation.

It's terribly different [now] for the young people. And, in a funny way, they got me. They taught me, made me conscious of things I'd put on the back burner. In the 1960s, a lot of young people came into AA, and at that point, I became sort of a reassuring presence, almost like a signpost in the group. They wanted to hear about my little six-year drinking career and my automobile accidents. My elitist background didn't matter to them.

Of course, in the 1960s everything became political. And my generation of gay people was very slow to get with the political thing, and very threatened by it at the beginning. The ones who were militant put me off terribly. I wasn't sympathetic. We all forged ahead in our fields, and the price was that everybody knew and nobody said. The first people out front—*[she stops]*. You just wanted to jump and hide! *I* did. If somebody was going to be caught out or make a scene, I wasn't going to be there for that. I thought, *Don't get any of that on me.*

The way I reacted isn't something I find attractive. I like courage! . . . So to be sort of republican about this is very antithetical. I've loathed snobs all my life and I've been a part of society where most of the people were snobbish. Though I was a maverick and very outspoken, I'd hide in the sand when I was vulnerable. I was very careful.

Could you say more about the 1960s, when there were gay militants around and you found yourself recoiling—

[Interrupting] I recoiled earlier. There were always militants, but the militants would be Radclyffe Hall—and I hate that book [Hall's 1928 novel *The Well of Loneliness*]! The only character I liked was the terrible society woman who set her up and then ran like a rabbit. That to me is understandable.

My mother was a very intelligent woman. She was what some people called a champagne socialist, the kind of woman who would stir things up. And in those days, to be for Roosevelt on the North Shore of Long Island was unheard of. She was very relieved when I joined AA. She came to one of the meetings and, oddly enough, Grace, or anyhow Maeve and Felicia were there. You must have heard Felicia's name.[4]

Maeve and Felicia were both very grand, and by grand I mean *[speaking slowly, in a low voice]* they "tahked like this: Some of us ah sickah than ahthahs," that kind of thing. Maeve was at NBC when I started there. She was very proud of me. She saw the fact that I was a woman [writer] as much more of a hurdle than I did early on. Growing up, we had women writers around the house all the time. I didn't know it was a bad thing.

In the 1950s, I went to the Caribbean with a man I was thinking of marrying, who was thinking of marrying me, although he was gay. I knew a lot more about him than he'd told me. I told him nothing about me. He didn't know until I suddenly appeared one day with this other woman.

It was terribly convenient. Suddenly you have this television executive, who was terrifying to everybody else, really on your side— picking up the check, making reservations, arranging where you were going to go. It was a great relief, this little romance.

When we went through customs, I noticed that he was a nervous wreck. I knew a man who'd received a dishonorable discharge because he was homosexual and I wondered if that kind of thing showed up on your passport. When we checked into the hotel, then it was my turn. I was as nervous as he'd been about the passport. I hated pretending to be married. . . . I hated pretending to be a couple when we weren't. I didn't want to say "we." It went against the grain to pretend to be something I wasn't. I thought I'd feel, *Whee! I'm one of them now!* But the pretense of being respectable wasn't fun. It was nerve-racking.

In the 1960s, I became part of a group of men and women who were all known to be what we were, where we were more or less accepted. A lot of us were very successful in our fields. We spent holidays and vacations together. We went to clubs and to gay bars. The first time I went to a gay bar, there was a cop outside. I was frightened, but my friend said, "They have to be there. They're paid off." That was the atmosphere we were in. The cop was paid off. He stood at the top of the stairs, and in a funny way, he was your protection.

One time I was at a bar, a fun one that had dancing, and the mob person who was really behind the scenes came in for a collection. There was some altercation between him and the woman who ran the bar, and he went away and got his mob. When they came back, one of them picked up a bar stool and threw it at the mirror behind the bar. We were all herded into a back office. I kept saying, "Why don't we call the police?" But my friend told me, "Never call the cops. Never!"

Do you understand what I'm saying? You were finally really in the underworld. Then *our* gangsters came to rescue us from the other gangsters—Don't ask! I don't know what the hell was going on! I do know that everyone who had a car, which was me—wheels, always. There was a guy assigned to us who followed us home so we'd be all right.

Did you find other gay people at meetings when you first came to AA?

Some of the guys would talk, at least to women. I did know, however one knew these things, that Marty Mann was said to be gay. That was very important to me. I'd heard her speak. She was very dynamic, very attractive, worldly. Again, the word is worldly. She was in the world. But she was also wearing twelve different hats. . . .

How did Marty manage to wear all of those hats? How did she find support?

Well, I think she finally had trouble, didn't she? I think she recovered herself, and that she was fine, but . . . I never knew about her slip at the time.

Did she connect with other gay people when she was traveling and lecturing?

[Exasperatedly] Yes! The network of gay people was *always* there. Like [Marty's affair with writer] Jane Bowles—that was a thing at one point I think. Bowles flew around and everybody was always trying to sober her up, quite futilely.

By the way, in case anybody cares, Bill Wilson had a mistress. I knew her very well. We went on a trip to Europe together with some other gay women, although she wasn't gay. She was there when Bill died.[5]

I once told her, "Helen, you ought to write a book."

"Oh, no!" she said. She practically had a heart attack at the thought!

"This isn't the royal family," I said. "He wasn't meant to be a saint." She was a wonderful speaker, too. Both of them were.

I think if I had anything in my mind, it was just a total, almost childlike insistence on keeping this one thing separate from everything else, so that it could never fail me, and I could never fail it, in any fundamental way—being in AA.

You kept being in AA separate from everything else?

Yes. Until the 1960s when one of my dearest friends became ill. Damien was a soul mate. I told him everything, and he told me everything. . . . Damien and his lover Emery started the Hetrick-Martin Institute.[6] He and Emery both died young.

Damien wrote me a letter: "I want you to know, before you find out from somebody else that I have AIDS." And at the same moment, my other best friend in life was smitten the same way. Alex was the art director at a publishing company. He looked like [Agatha Christie's detective Hercule] Poirot—dapper, the mustache, the Man About Town. . . . Alex . . . never said the word "AIDS." He died first.

You couldn't go see him because he didn't want to see you. Finally, one was allowed to know, when he landed in St. Vincent's Hospital, and it was the AIDS floor. Then he broke down and cried in my arms, this man who never admitted he had AIDS. I just grabbed him and held him while he cried. *[We sit quietly.]*

It's hard to cross the gap of the years. People don't know what you're talking about half the time. And what looked like cowardice—was—it was how to survive. I can't imagine I'd ever play it very differently. You go along, and you finally find something, and someone, who—and you think, *If you don't like it you can go screw yourself!* I—and I'm told now I'm a pioneer—well, a very strange one.

[After a few moments, I ask] Pucky, have you ever been to a gay AA meeting?

Oh yes, I've spoken at them. I loved it, and they liked me. I was the last man standing at one of them once.[7] . . .

Do you happen to know of the three women who met with Bill Wilson in 1945 to talk about starting an AA meeting for homosexuals in New York?

I'm afraid not. Marty might have been one of them. But I don't think she would have been for starting a gay meeting. Marty's anonymity was a big issue back then.[8]

Arlene Francis had a talk show. She knew I was in AA and that I'd done "Drink like a Lady" for [the 1960s' television series] *The Defenders,* which she loved. She'd say, *"Why* won't you come on my show and say you're in AA?" She was dying for me to do it. I told her I couldn't.

You're out front; everyone thinks you're wonderful, and a saint. Then something goes wrong, and you're not wonderful anymore. You drag down the sides, so to speak. It's a weight, a burden. It's like people sidling up to you and telling you how much willpower you have, when you know sobriety has nothing to do with willpower. Willpower is what makes you keep going on other things, but not this.

One last question. Have you had any heroes in your recovery?

I looked up to my father in a way; he was a charming, gentle, funny man. He made every attempt to reach you that could be made by somebody who was themselves unreachable. Damien, certainly, Bud and Marty, and, God knows, Bill, because he was brilliant. There was also a friend at *Harper's Bazaar* who joined AA. She had a terrible slip and went her own way. She broke my heart. I saw her once. She'd lost all the teeth on one side. And I once saw that little Ebby person. It was the first time I ever went to the AA dinner. Bill Wilson spoke, and coming out of the hall, I saw a little man on the street outside, like a drunk in the movies, yelling, "Lemme at him! Lemme at him!"

He was drunk?

Yes! Pissed! He's yelling, "Aaah! He thinks *he* started it. I started it. *I* started it!"[9]

It's an illness. As Felicia and Maeve were always saying, "Some of us ah sickah than ahthahs." Well, some of us are luckier than others are. I think luck plays a part and, God knows, attendance at meetings. . . . But, drunk or sober, they are all friends of the heart.

L. B.

[L. B. got sober in New York in 1953. She is an addiction medicine specialist, now retired. She is currently active in an animal rescue organization.]

I started going to AA about a year before I got sober, so that would make it 1952. I was living in Greenwich Village and knew quite a lot of gay and lesbian people. My drinking buddy was pressuring me to go to AA and I was insisting that I didn't need it, so I decided I would shut him up by demanding something I knew he couldn't produce.

"Okay," I told him, "I'll go to AA, provided you find someone to take me who is a woman roughly my age, smarter than me, Jewish, and lesbian," which is not as dumb as it sounds. I'd left the Catholic Church with a great deal of anger in early adolescence, and I was pretty sure that a good Jewish liberal from New York would not try to shut me back into Mother Church. I had read somewhere that Jews didn't get alcoholism, and I had also been told that gays and lesbians did not successfully get sober. I knew there couldn't be any women in AA roughly my age, and certainly not one smarter than me, so that clinched that. The trouble was that within seventy-two hours [AA] had found her.

Lila was working for Marty Mann at the National Council on Alcoholism at the time. Not only did Lila meet my criteria, she came complete with a lot of information about alcoholism that the average AA sponsor would not have had. She dropped a whole packet of pamphlets on me that I was to read, and I devoured them with great interest. Mind you, I had no intention of going to AA. For several months, I made excuses for why I could and would not go. Later when I hit bottom, with a terrible crash, I still had Lila's name and phone number and I called her. And I've been sober since.

Did you meet other lesbians or gay men in AA?

Yes, but that was because of Lila. There was a small handful of gay and lesbian people who would discuss which meetings to go to, and the same little group would turn up at those meetings. There was also a young people's AA group in Manhattan that Barry L. and Damien

M. went to. Damien later got back in my life because his lover Emery was a psychiatrist at the same hospital where I practiced.

Emery and Damien started the Hetrick-Martin Institute. Kids were being kicked out of their homes in all kinds of places. They'd get off the bus at the Port Authority Terminal, where they'd find some charming gentleman saying, "Do you have a place to stay tonight, Sonny?" and pretty soon Sonny was turning tricks, hooked on drugs, and in all kinds of trouble.

It was very difficult for Damien and Emery because, at the time, any man showing an interest in gay youth was obviously a pedophile. But they bit the bullet and salvaged the kids they could. They subsequently formed the Harvey Milk High School—*[A furious barking suddenly erupts in the background, accompanied by the scrabbling of tiny feet trying to gain traction on a hard floor.]*

I don't know if I told you, but we do dog rescue *[rurruuhr]*—Stop! *[Rruh!]* That's our three-pound Butch. She's a very small Butch, but she's all muscle.

What kind of dog is she?

They're all Chihuahuas. She's sitting here with a bone in her mouth wearing an Elizabethan collar because she's recently had eye surgery. Nancy was trying to take a picture of her so Butch immediately started swearing *[rrruhh!]. [I hear a door open and close, and the barking slowly grows fainter and subsides.]*

You were talking about Damien and Emery, and that, at meetings like the young people's group, you had gay people around you in AA.

Yes. It wasn't a very large group because there weren't many young people in AA at the time; it got the dwindles rather quickly. When you have a small population for an AA group, it has to be carefully nurtured or everything comes apart, particularly if it's a group that's not going to welcome anybody and everybody.

Were you out to many people?

At that time I was. I was certainly out to myself. Most of us at the time were not particularly out to the world at large. I was out to other gay and lesbian people, okay?[10]

Did you attend any gay meetings when they started? Were they helpful?

I can't say I found them to be any more helpful than regular meetings. They were a better place to meet people to socialize with, but that was not my primary motive for going to AA in the first place. I can say one thing strong and clear: I would much rather be at any women's AA meeting, whether there are lesbians there or not, than in a meeting with both men and women where I have to listen to the men holding forth endlessly and the women not speaking up.

You have worked with many recovering alcoholics in your career. Is there anything you have discovered about gay and lesbian alcoholics, in particular?

Well, first off, that there are an awful lot of us. We have a culture that gives us every opportunity to develop alcoholism and other addictions, if we have any talent for it in the first place. Nobody has the stats, so you don't have to worry about that too much, though everybody has opinions, but, certainly, we have our fair share. So there have always been plenty of gay and lesbian people around, both as patients and people we could use to help patients.

Have you discovered anything about yourself as a gay alcoholic, working with other gay alcoholics?

I'm not quite sure how to answer that. That's more the question that comes up with any person in recovery working in this field, the disclosure question. One of the big arguments, always, if you're working with alcoholics, is whether or not to tell them you're in AA. Do you talk "we," or do you talk "I" and "you"? My feeling is that it's good to have individuals on the treatment staff who can play different roles. So if I'm playing doctor—a heavy with a white coat and a stethoscope—I/You is a better role for me than being the curiosity, the Woman Doctor. So as a doctor, I would be the I/You person and let the counselors be the We.

There is a certain mystique in being a doctor. It goes with the costume, the idea that doctors know more than other people, which is nonsense. The idea that anyone with a medical education is an authority. You know better, I know better, if you've lived a life, but the point is that patients believe it, and they will accept stuff from a doctor that they will not accept from an AA sponsor. The challenge is to use that as best you can on the patient's behalf.

You certainly don't need to get into self-indulgent confessionals about your own story. Patients don't really give a damn about you anyway. They just want to get comfortable, and out of trouble, without making any changes in their lives. *[We have a good laugh over that last statement.]*

L___, I'd like to ask you about the foreword you wrote in 1995 to a special issue of the Journal of Gay and Lesbian Social Services *titled "Addiction and Recovery of Gay and Lesbian Persons." In it, you describe being at a gathering of physicians and other alcoholism professionals in New York in the early 1950s and hearing someone say, "Many people can recover from alcoholism. Except, of course, the homosexuals." What was it like to hear that, and why did people believe that homosexuals could not recover?*

First of all, an awful lot of people didn't know a homosexual if they fell over one. You know that this was at a time when most of us were pretty closeted. Barry and I were both in the room, and we were busy trying not to catch each other's eye when the statement was made, and there was another gay man in the room who was sort of looking at the ceiling while this psychiatrist held forth about her theories. My guess is that what she was saying was that in her experience, this was the case, and with those attitudes, I'm not surprised that her patients never recovered. She was probably reporting very accurately what she['d] found, poor dear!

I think an awful lot of the reasoning back then was that we were drinking *because* we were gay and lesbian. If we refused to stop that nonsense and straighten out, and have heterosexual marriages and kids then, clearly, we weren't well. And therefore couldn't be expected to stop drinking.

Now we are able to see these as totally different things. I can be alcoholic, I can be lesbian, I can have pneumonia, I can have breast cancer, I can have blue eyes, [and] they can all go together. But they're not necessarily causally related.

I assume there was a point at which you were in the closet professionally. Is that correct?

I was pretty much out of the closet professionally at my first job. I was a librarian for the New York Public Library for five or six years and there were plenty of lesbian librarians around, though we didn't talk about it. On the other hand, I didn't feel uncomfortable or that I needed to hide who I was, because I knew perfectly well that the woman who ran the library lived on West 8th Street and had a female lover. We didn't discuss it; I just knew it.

Later when I decided I wanted to go to medical school, I thought I had trouble enough being an alcoholic and being thirty years old without hitting them over the head with, "Guess what. I'm a dyke!" So I went back into my closet, tidied it up nicely, and concentrated on being a reliable hardworking pre-med student. Long after that— when I was strong enough professionally, and could do pretty much what I damn well chose and get away with it, I became much more casual about being out. And after I retired, now I'm completely out.

I am trying to learn more about Barry L. Would you tell me a little about your acquaintance?

For someone I knew as many years as I knew Barry, I can't give you much detail. I knew Barry initially as someone who attended meetings with me. I met him early on, together with his lover Spencer who was in Al-Anon. He was well known around the [AA] General Service Office where he did a lot of the writing for the book *Living Sober.* He did a variety of things. I hired him as an alcoholism counselor when I was getting started at Smithers [Alcoholism Treatment and Training Center at Roosevelt Hospital in New York]. At that time, he was very interested in writing articles for the *AA Grapevine.*

We did a little article together on the growth and size of AA as estimated by the increase in the number of groups. If you figured that 80 to 90 percent of groups that were supposed to report to General Service in fact did so, and that each group represented perhaps fifteen or twenty people, you could do a quick and dirty estimate of the number of alcoholics that were AA members. Of course, AA groups have rarely been willing to report; they've been wonderfully cavalier about that.[11]

But we did the article and we even ran across a rather interesting phenomenon. If you graphed the increase in the number of groups, for a time the growth was almost linear and then suddenly it would plateau and then become linear again. We thought, *Hmm, something's going on here,* and Barry tracked it down. It seems that some of the early AAs had been lying about how many AAs there were! When it came out that the honesty part of the program was not being very well observed at the General Service Office, the decision was made to just shut up about it and use the numbers they had, until reality caught up with those numbers, and then start plotting growth again. We don't have that in our article, but you'll see some of it in there.

Was the article published in the AA Grapevine?

No, the *International Journal of the Addictions,* or the *British Journal of the Addictions.* You could probably track it down if you wanted to look up my papers at the Archives of Women in Medicine in Philadelphia. I would say they have easily 90 percent of what I've written, should anybody ever wish to find them and make me immortal.

I am always glad to hear that someone has left her papers to an organization that will preserve them and make them accessible to others.

The Archives of Women in Medicine primarily wants first physicians—the first black one, the first Native American one—the ones who have been presidents of the American Medical Women's Association over the years. They also want people who have received the Elizabeth Blackwell Award. The day I won that one, they decided they wanted everything that I'd ever written.[12]

In closing, could you describe some of the ways being a sober lesbian today is different from how it was when you first came into AA?

It is a completely different world. When I was first trying to find out about gay and lesbian people in high school, I went to the dictionaries and the encyclopedias and I couldn't find anything, except dreary psychiatric texts like *Psychopathia Sexualis,*[13] things like that. We had gone from simply being wicked, and needing to be burned at the stake, to being sick and needing to be fixed by psychiatrists. The myth was that we were very strange people and that there weren't very many of us.

Today I can walk into almost any bookstore and find two or three *shelves,* if it's a big bookstore, on gay and lesbian stuff. And if I want to take the trouble to subscribe to *Out* magazine, or *The Advocate,* or a variety of other sheets, I can do that. I can track down the presses that tell me lots of stuff about me. I can find therapists who will not try and fix me. I can even choose a gay therapist, if I want to. It's a much more open, accepting society.

Lois P.

[Lois got sober in New York in 1959. Since the early 1970s, she and her partner Helen have spent their summers in Cherry Grove, a gay community established on Fire Island in New York in the late 1930s. I spoke with Lois by phone at their winter home in Florida.]

In 1959, I went to Ohio to visit my family at Christmastime and I was drunk for about a week. Christmas dinner went on for hours, and the food, which all my life had been wonderful, I could barely look at. I came back to New York City and continued to drink until I could no longer hold anything down. I got sicker and sicker, and I began to hallucinate.[14] I heard music that would not stop, the death scenes from operas—*Lucia di Lammermoor, La Traviata*—all that stuff, which I used to play constantly, and cry.

My lover came in. "Oh my god," she said, "I have to get help. I'm going to call AA!" and she made the call.

The AA person on the phone tells her, "I have to speak to the drunk," so she says to me, lying in the bed, "They have to talk to the drunk."

Well, this was very jarring to my nerves [being called a drunk].

I went to the phone and they said they'd send someone to see me. This was right after New Year's in New York, when AA was very busy in the city, and appearing at my door some hours later were two black men. The older man was sober seven or eight years; he was a minister. He'd brought the young guy with him to see what alcoholics look like when they're in bad shape. Having had no contact with AA, I assumed that everyone in AA was male and black.[15]

They came in and the older man says to my roommate, "Go out and buy her two beers. She's going to go into convulsions." So she came back with two cans of beer and gave me one. She drank the other one. I sipped on it and shook and shook and shook. All the while, this man is looking at me with love and understanding. He said, "I feel that pain shooting up your spine and hitting the back of your head." It was an amazing first identification of one drunk to another.

I asked him about AA. "What kind of money does it cost to join?"

"No money."

"Do I have to get on a mailing list?"

"No mailing list."

He took out the AA Preamble and read it. I'd never heard such a thing! I was a health and phys ed teacher so I knew a little bit about agencies, but nothing about AA. "I'll have a woman call you," he said. "Maybe you'd like to go to a meeting." She called and we made arrangements to meet at a meeting. I saw her two or three times; she was very kind and helpful.

I went to the Morningside Group in Manhattan, which would be considered a low-bottom group, a very low bottom for this arrogant teacher, you see. I thought, *Well, they're not drinking, but that's all I can say for them.* I stayed dry for two months. The last drunk ended March 7, 1960, and I have been sober since.

I had not definitely decided that I would live a homosexual life. I thought this was a temporary condition [, that] one could will oneself in and out of this. That was the belief then, that homosexuals were emotionally retarded, that they hadn't grown up yet and matured into being heterosexual. So when I told my sponsor who came to see me after the last binge that I was a lesbian—and I did tell her—I was too drunk and sick to play games, and if she was going to help me, I wanted her to know what the score was.

"Okay," she said, "but if I were you I'd keep it to yourself." That was her advice.

In my third or fourth year [of sobriety], I fell in love. And though that relationship didn't work out, I thought, *I am going to stop playing games with myself.* I was dating men and had had relationships and sex with some of them, but I could no longer blame it on them being bad lovers or that I just hadn't found the right one. I realized that I was a lesbian and that I wanted women.

I went to Greenwich Village and decided that was where and how I was going to live, to live openly—not professionally, but personally, and in AA—as a lesbian. Greenwich Village is a liberal place. There are all kinds there. "Yes, she's one of those too" was the attitude, with very little judgment. So I had that. The rest of the world had not changed, of course. But I had a sense of freedom in my personal life, in AA, and in me.

There were two very active, primarily gay groups in New York at the time, both in churches. We had slang names for them—one we called the Red Door, the other we called the Saturday Night Follies—because everyone went there more for social activity than for AA, and that's where I met a lot of people. We socialized in meetings, during coffee hours, after meetings, in each other's homes. It was a great life! The Greenwich Village Group, one of the original AA groups, was mixed [gay and straight], and Perry Street was always mixed. At Perry Street, there were twenty to twenty-five meetings a week.

I found the men were the biggest help to me in AA because there was no sexual attraction between us, so I could be open and frank without getting involved with crushes. That was a problem for me from the very beginning and sometimes still is, and I'm seventy-two years old! It took me quite awhile to realize my motivations, and that I'd better clean up my act. . . . I've found sponsoring another lesbian to be a hazardous business most of the time. In AA they say men sponsor men and women sponsor women, but I firmly believe that with us, at least in the early stages [of sobriety], women need men sponsors and men need women sponsors.

Did you know Barry L.? Can you tell me anything about him?

Barry was a dear friend of mine. I was thinking of going into [the field of] alcoholism and Barry was an avid developer of professionals in AA. He was a lay therapist, one of the first I knew.[16] He was very close to Marty Mann, and Dr. Ruth Fox, and others who formed the National Council on Alcoholism [NCA]. With his encouragement, I took an NCA course on leadership and professionalism, and got a master's degree in public health. Barry helped me through all that because I had various blocks.

We were sitting in a restaurant one day and I said, "Barry, I can't write."

He handed me a napkin and a pencil and said, "Put that down."

"Put what down?"

"[Put down] 'I can't write.'" So I wrote it on the napkin.

"There. You just did."

Just like that, whatever it is you're thinking, that's what you put on paper, which is an instant example of, *Of course I can write, so what's all this bullshit, "I can't write"?*

I was horrified when he became ill. He was one of the first of our dear friends that went. From then on life changed. *[She falls silent.]*

AIDS hit that crowd and our friends on Fire Island like a medieval plague. Some of them you saw one day and a week later, they'd died of pneumonia. Or they developed this awful cancer-type thing that no one could identify. It was horrible. Barry was the first on that. I still miss him—him and a whole group of others. *[We sit quietly.]*

[Sighing deeply] I can sit on the deck of our house on Fire Island and look to each side, and across the way, and all the way up and down the street. They all went, and not well. They were young, strong men and they did not die easily. People are still dying. The awful thing about it is that it's as if it never existed. They've gone back to the old behavior. Not good.

In 1968, I began teaching at the University of New York. I had my opportunity to teach a course in public health to budding social workers. . . . I wrote the course and taught it for over twenty years, as well as courses in drugs and alcohol, women's health issues, and human sexuality. *[Chuckling]* So, I ended up a college professor!

In my human sexuality course, if a student wanted to talk about their sexuality they could. As the teacher I forbid anyone to ridicule or to judge. If someone was homophobic, I'd say, "You believe that, and I don't question it and I don't judge it, but I expect you to develop a similar attitude toward other people."

When teaching, I remained anonymous regarding my sexuality. If someone pressed me, I'd say, "Nowhere on the course outline does it say, 'And now we will talk about Professor P____'s sex life.'" Oh, they would get furious!

"That's not being honest," some would say. It was honest. It may have been evasive, but it was honest. Because you and I both know that there's a segment of people's minds that when they find out you're a lesbian everything you say is filtered through it. It distorts the whole picture. So I didn't permit it to be brought up. I had a lot of fun with it, really. Most students would change by the time they walked out. They'd be more open-minded and gentle about it. It was an amazing transformation, but it took a lot of patience.

I understand that you've sponsored many people in AA over the years. Would you talk a little about that experience?

The majority of gays have a torturous experience with the Fourth Step, as I did myself. There is a lot of fear about being who we are, and the fear is associated with violence—verbal and physical violence. This isn't as prevalent now as it used to be but, in those days, to approach the Fourth Step was very difficult. Almost every person whose Fourth Step I listened to had been violated in some way: rapes, beatings, being institutionalized, being forced to stay in an institution until one was cured of homosexuality, shock treatments. When I got into the Fourth Step with individuals, it would be very painful.

People would become hysterical just from their own fear. A lot of people would give me their Fourth Steps and then not talk to me! They were so ashamed of what they had told me, and so fearful of what I would do with the information.

And I would try very hard, as they were telling me these most intimate things, to share my own, to match in severity what I had done and experienced, or what was done to me, so they'd get what we were talking about. So I had an opportunity as well, because there were some things I was holding back too. In the end, both of us were washed pretty clean.

I was the youngest of four children with a brutal father. For some reason I rebelled against him, and it worked. I felt empowered by that. I spent my entire youth and adulthood coming up with defenses against attack. A lot of this is just dumb luck, or guidance, or an angel on the shoulder, however you want to look at it, but I moved through various dangerous situations without being hurt. Sometimes it was deviousness, sometimes it was compliance to a certain extent, and sometimes it was attack. It's instinctual with me to protect myself.

When I went into that classroom, I had no guidelines on how to deal with the subject of being a lesbian, but somehow, the guidance was there, and it worked. I'm not quite sure where this comes from, but AA has helped tremendously. Whenever that feeling comes over me, *Uh oh, this is dangerous—watch out,* I think, *Upp!* And go calm. I ask for guidance, for direction, and it comes.

This is a message a lot of alcoholics are grateful to hear. "Let go. Let God do this." And once they try it, they see that it works beautifully, if you can really let go. Don't manipulate it; don't think about it. Just let it go. *[Laughing]* If you do nothing else, you'll shut up!

I go to an AA group here [in Florida] at the Hillsborough Pines Club. I go to this group because it is completely mixed, with gays in the minority. There are homophobes in there, and they can be vicious. I just look at them and smile.

There's a man in the meeting who's taken an attraction to me. He's older, like me. He's had cancer, like me. He has hearing aids, like me. He is explicitly well mannered, and he keeps trying to get me to go out with him, to have coffee, to go to the movies, all this sort of thing. Well, last night he started again, and I hadn't seen him in five months! I thought, *Surely he knows.*

"Earle, stop trying to date me. I'm a lesbian."

"I—Er, you? You're a lesbian? I didn't—I never—"

"Why not?"

"Because—because you're not nasty. I've found that gay people are mean and nasty—hostile."

"Oh," I say.

"Well, you're so nice."

I sat there quietly. After, I saw that I'd shocked the hell out of him. I asked for direction.

"You married?" he says.

"Yes. Same woman, twenty-eight years."

"Wow," [he says].

After the meeting I told him I was sorry that I'd come on so strong because I knew I'd shocked him.

Then he says, "You know, something happened to me when I was younger. Can I talk to you about it sometime? It still bothers me."

I got quiet inside. Then I said, "Here's my phone number. Give me a call." We'll see what happens.

So, outside of what has been my life in metropolitan New York and on Fire Island, this still exists. We bring a lot of crap on ourselves when we get in a hostile environment.

I heard that Marty M. and Priscilla P. founded the AA group on Fire Island. Do you know when it began?

I first attended the Cherry Grove Group in 1973. They had just started meeting at the firehouse when I started going; it had been at Bob B.'s house [before that]. They hadn't wanted to meet in a public facility before then because they wanted to be anonymous. Now we had a public entrance into a community building which meant a sign up front, and all this stuff.

Ah, the double stigma at work. I've been studying the ways gay groups protected themselves from homophobia in the AA community. Now here's an example of an AA group in a gay community protecting its members from the stigma of alcoholism.

We developed a silent reputation, as AA has for so many years, of protecting each other's anonymity. You don't want other people to know you're alcoholic until you're secure in your sobriety. There are nine meetings a week in that firehouse now. There's very little discussion of being gay at those meetings. We're all gay, so what's the big deal? *[She laughs.]* This is why I say I need *some* contact with the real world!

Lesbians have been publicly shamed at meetings here [in Florida]. There are very few people who do that, but they are here. Anyone who knows anything about where I come from and where I go in summer knows I'm gay, and some people just leave it at that. I have a neighbor who wants to get out of me that Helen and I are lovers. I get so pissed at her that I won't say it. I told her, "What we do here is nobody's business."

Now, if I were a modern-day lesbian, I would get out my banner and stomp up and down the street saying, "I am what I am and you have to accept it!" I no longer feel that way. You don't have to accept it and I don't have to accept you. It's a live-and-let-live attitude, which I am well schooled to accept. When I see others doing this, I think, *We need this lunatic fringe to change society,* but I am too old to take up another torch, to tell you the truth. So that's the way it is.

This is good for my humility, because if I took up the torch it would turn into some grandiose battle. It's like justified anger. I no longer have the nervous system to take the battering that goes with it. You can't eradicate hate. . . .

It sounds to me like you are creating change in your own way. Like with Earle.

I look at it from the angle that says, "Oh, I wish you would learn what I have learned!" They don't know what they're missing! We are wonderful people *[laughing]* once we grow up! Every once in a while someone's house is trashed, or their car tires are deflated, and I think, *Well, that's part of it, I guess.* When I go home to Ohio, it's the same thing. The only way I can make my sister comfortable is to not talk about it at all. And it isn't necessarily her. It's her husband, her children, their neighbors, all that stuff.

Someone mentioned to me that you are black.

No, that's [my partner] Helen. Do you recall the section about racism in Esther Newton's book about Cherry Grove?[17] She mentioned that Helen was the first black woman to own a house there. Can you believe it? The first black woman to own a house in Cherry Grove was in 1983! We have our own prejudices within the gay community. Helen has a unique way of blending in. You can always tell when someone is surprised. They usually say, "You speak so *well,* Helen." It's awful.

Do you have any heroes you've looked up to in sobriety?

When I was newly sober, I'd get all rattled, and I'd call my sponsor who'd say, "Lois, God will take care of you," which is true, as it has occurred for all these years. Whenever I am very upset, that phrase still comes to mind. And there's a man named Ed, who ended up a trustee of Alcoholics Anonymous. He had a sense of humor that was absolutely irreverent. Ed was able to turn the saddest situations into laughter. In tragedy, laughter of all things is the most healing. I saw how valuable laughter was and I've nurtured it—not only in AA but also in my life, and in the classroom. There is such a distance between ridicule and the genuine healing laughter of AA. It is one of the greatest gifts I've been given. Bless his soul for being in my life. He's now passed of AIDS. I seek out people who have the kind of humor Ed had.

And of course, there was Barry. He believed I had the ability to do what I did, despite all my hangups, despite the missing areas of my life because I was drunk through my twenties. To this day, it is still amazing to me! In the home I grew up in, if you were not smiling and willing to be a housekeeper—and I was not—you were ruined. I had no examples. I had no role models to do what I did. AA gave me a way of life that worked. Thank you, Alcoholics Anonymous, and all the people in it.

I was fourteen years sober before I spoke to a group of lesbians in Alcoholics Anonymous, and I was so frightened I started to shiver. I think the fear was about talking to my own people. We all know each other here, right? We know each other right down to the bedroom, and I was frightened to expose myself. And when I spoke at that meeting, the same thing happened that happened [here], when I spoke here last week.

[I was asked to speak and] I had just five minutes notice. I started to think, *Here we go again. Say this in a certain way, so you don't tell them you're—I wonder if I should—Upp! No. Just open your mouth and let it come out.*

As the Preamble is being read I pray, "Please God, let me say what needs to be said in this room," and it's just amazing what happens. I say things I would *never* think of saying! Have you ever been used as an instrument? I don't know it while it's happening, but I know it when it's finished.

I noticed there was a newcomer at the meeting and that gave me direction to tell the end of my drinking story. My last drunk involved a violent dyke drama, believe me. This fight occurred between me and my lover over booze. It was like that awful scene in *Days of Wine and*

Roses where everything goes insane. All the violence is being done to me, because I'm too drunk to lash out. My mouth is going. I'm throwing stuff out the window of a twelve-story building and slashing fur coats. Finally she knocks me unconscious with a perfume bottle. And as it's hitting my head I think, *You idiot. Is this how you have to learn? You* are *insane. Your life* is *unmanageable. Get back to AA. And this time, listen.*

That was my introduction. And as I'm telling this story, because it is what came to mind, I wasn't concerned [about changing pronouns], about "he," or "she," or "it," or anything else. *Okay kids. Here it is!* And once again, after the meeting I got that affirmation—the arms coming around me, the hugs—from the straights, from this, and from that. I thought, *Finally, I am free.*

We've lived here in Florida for five years. Living in a completely gay community and then coming down here [in winter] and facing the real world, the realization comes that we are not liberated. I can't expect that in my lifetime, but I can be an example that's positive. I'm surrounded by straight people—I'm talking about the neighbors—and they have accepted us. If it hadn't been for AA, I think my innate hostility about being judged probably would have interfered with that. I would have made remarks. I would not have been able to reach out or respond when they asked for help: "Could you water my flowers while we're away?"

The important thing is that being gay is not an issue with me. I am what I am. Helen gets horrified, because she's a classy lady and I have a tendency to be outrageous. I go out in the morning to let the dog take a pee and pick up the paper in my pajamas, and she gives me a look. But if you think I'm going to get dressed and put on makeup just to walk the dog and pick up the newspaper, you are sadly mistaken. *[Grinning]* But now *she's* doing it!

Gay AA in Boston, 1949

Although it is little more than a historical sketch, I feel that it is important to include Ed S.'s account of the first gay AA group in Boston, Massachusetts, in this chapter. His remarks are excerpted from a recording made at a workshop at the International AA Convention in 1980. To provide some additional context for his story, I've sketched in a few details of my own, before and after the material presented from the tape.

In the 1940s, membership in AA grew rapidly. In the spring of 1947, Marty M. had delivered a speech about alcoholism and AA to a crowd of 700 at Boston's Brown Hall. According to a note about the event in the *AA Grapevine,* police and firemen had had to turn away an additional 300 people who'd come to hear her presentation ("S.R.O. for AA" 1947).

At that time, the AA Central Service Committee of Boston, who'd sponsored Marty's talk, was also hosting a series of noontime discussions so that people in Boston who were interested in AA could find out what was happening in the organization. They had invited Bill Wilson up from New York on several occasions to talk.

The Twelve Traditions were not formally adopted by AA until 1950, although Bill had been speaking and writing about them for some time. In the 1940s, there was a great deal of confusion in AA about how AA was supposed to work. A particularly thorny issue concerned who was eligible to join AA, and different groups had widely varying rules for membership.

> In those days we were always talking about the mythical character called the pure alcoholic; no complications, you understand, just a guzzler. We actually thought we were like that ourselves! Hence, when members began pouring in, our worry mounted. "Won't there be mighty queer people? Won't there be criminals? Won't there be social undesirables?" we asked. Mixed with a certain amount of snobbishness and smugness, this was downright fear.[18]

> Bill Wilson
> On the history of the Third Tradition
> *Alcoholics Anonymous Comes of Age: A Brief History of A.A.* (1957)

In 1949, a handful of gay men who were staying sober in Boston AA gathered in a rooming house on Beacon Hill. They talked again that evening about what it might be like to have an AA meeting "for our kind." Thirty years later, Ed S. gave this account of their activities, and the first gay AA group in Boston.

Ed S.

In those days, as it was explained in the Third Tradition, I was a queer. It's printed that way: "Queer." . . . But I didn't have anywhere else to go. And I came back [to AA] in 1945.

But . . . I did it the hard way—because I could find sobriety, but I couldn't find serenity. I couldn't reach out to the people who could understand me, as I wanted to be understood, who I could share my heartbreak with and my happiness—more than just sobriety.

I was transferred to Philadelphia with my job, which entailed traveling up and down the entire East Coast. The young man I was staying with, who I'd met in Biloxi many years before was living with me, and we were considered—you whispered it in those days—lovers. But he had a friend in Boston, and this friend had other friends. We felt comfortable with them because they were in the fellowship, too.

[But] there was nothing much we could do about it, except sit on Myrtle Street, in back of the State House in Boston, and talk to each other about how nice it was to be sober. But wasn't it awful to be queer, in staid old Boston? The year was 1949.

I had seen Bill Wilson in a brown bagger lunch. The office workers used to run in, chomp on their sandwiches, and listen intently to what sobriety was all about, in a sort of AA Roundup, a workshop, in those days.

These gentlemen from Boston—Skip and Buzz were their names—Clyde would sit in the background, [as] he was a shy sort of thing—said to me, "Why don't you, seeing as how you know who Bill Wilson is, and you have talked to him, why don't you go up and ask him whether we could have a special group just for ourselves, just for our kind?"

I was hesitant, because I wasn't completely honest [about my homosexuality], and I didn't know how to be completely honest, in a fellowship that only had "pure alcoholics" in the beginning, but who were trying to reach out. We argued amongst ourselves about what we should do.

"Let's draw straws," they said, and I drew the first straw. "That's the shortest, that's the shortest!" they said. "You have to go!"

Well, I've got to tell you that I'm shaking up here on this stage right now, but you never saw anything like the way I was shaking then. It was midway between now and the DTs of the LaSalle State Hospital.

I approached the great man. "Bill, my name is Ed, and we have a problem. And we would like to start a specialty group, or something special, in Boston AA."

I could see by the pained expression on his face that he had been beleaguered by many specialty things, and that he had a lot of things on his mind.

"What kind of a specialty group?" he said.

I don't know how I got out that long word. *[Speaking slowly]* "H-o-m-o-s-e-x-u-a-l."

"Now, just a minute," Bill said. "Let's not go any farther. Are these people alcoholic?"

"Yes."

And he said, "Whatever you do to discuss your problems, and to stay sober, if you will go to any lengths to achieve sobriety, please do so."

So in 1949, queer AA came to Boston.

The group per se was probably doomed from the very beginning, because right across from this little father-son-holy-ghost house[18] was the Stag Hotel. "Men Only" it said. We met there, and there were a lot of distractions, as you might well imagine. But the group did survive for the years that I knew of. . . . That was the nuclei. That seed was planted on the East Coast, as best I know.

Postscript

Men's rooming houses and residential hotels have fostered gay friendships and communities in American cities for decades (Chauncey 1994). Ed jokes that the members of this early meeting were too distracted by sexual pursuits to sustain the group for very long, but it is more likely that their meeting succumbed to an increasingly hostile social climate and the rise of McCarthyism in the 1950s.

The Stag Hotel, built at the turn of the century, was originally a well-appointed rooming house called Beacon Chambers. Over the years, the building slowly fell into disrepair, and in the 1970s, a fire closed the old hotel. Today, a newly renovated and restored Beacon

Chambers stands at 19 Myrtle Street, where it provides modern apartments for elderly, disabled, and low-income residents of Boston. And on Friday nights, the How It Works Group of Boston holds a Big Book study there.

Chapter 5

Finding AA:
Groups, Directories,
and the First Gay AA Meeting

Introduction

When the first gay Alcoholics Anonymous groups started trying to register with their local service offices, and with the AA General Service Office (GSO) in New York, they sparked a growing controversy in Alcoholics Anonymous. In the late 1960s and early 1970s the idea of gay people publicizing a gathering of any kind was unheard of. To understand what happened, it will be useful to take a brief look at the different kinds of AA meetings that are held, and how AA group directories are published and used.

The debates at the General Service Conference that followed the appearance of the first gay meetings were framed by the issue of whether or not there ought to be "special purpose groups" in AA. The exact definition of an AA group—what it was, and what it was not— was also central to these discussions, and a lengthy and painstaking reexamination of this topic was launched. That issue was to be resolved years later, long after the controversy over gay groups had passed.

Simply put, an AA group is a collection of alcoholics who meet regularly for the purpose of holding an AA meeting. But there are countless variations on this basic theme. AA's *World Directory,* the list of registered groups published by the AA General Service Office in New York, offers this definition:

The History of Gay People in Alcoholics Anonymous
Published by The Haworth Press, Inc., 2007. All rights reserved.
doi:10.1300/5699_05

Our membership ought to include all who suffer from alcoholism. Hence, we may refuse none who wish to recover. Nor ought AA membership ever depend upon money or conformity. Any two or three alcoholics gathered together for sobriety may call themselves an AA group, provided that, as a group, they have no other affiliation. Each Alcoholics Anonymous group ought to be a spiritual entity having but one primary purpose—that is carrying its message to the alcoholics who still suffer. (Alcoholics Anonymous 2002)

Types of Meetings

Most AA meetings begin with the Serenity Prayer and what's known as "the AA Preamble," which provides a short description of the program. This is followed by a reading from the fifth chapter of *Alcoholics Anonymous* ("How It Works"), which includes a reading of the Twelve Steps.

There are many different types of meetings in AA. There are women's meetings, men's meetings, beginners' meetings, and meditation meetings. There are meetings for young people, old people, gay people, and people of color. There are smoking meetings and nonsmoking meetings. There are meetings held in languages other than English, and meetings interpreted for the hearing impaired. At speaker/discussion meetings, the kind most frequently depicted in movies and TV programs, a member tells his or her AA story and suggests a topic for discussion. At Big Book and Step Study meetings, AA literature is read and discussed, usually *Alcoholics Anonymous* or *Twelve Steps and Twelve Traditions,* a collection of essays by Bill Wilson. At a chip meeting, you can pick up a token with your length of sobriety printed on it and a hearty round of applause.

AA groups convene in church basements, community centers, office buildings, hospitals, treatment centers, and prisons. Many meet in "Alano clubs," facilities where meetings are offered throughout the day. (Alano clubs are operated by AA members, not by Alcoholics Anonymous.) Meetings start at dawn, noon, midnight, and nearly every hour in between.

Some groups meet once a week; others meet every day. For example, Honolulu's Twelve Coconuts Group meets every morning at 7:00

a.m. on Waikiki Beach beneath a stand of coconut trees. In San Francisco, the Bushwackers Group meets on Saturdays for a simultaneous meeting and a hike. (The schedule notes that the Bushwackers hold an "easier, softer hike" on the first Saturday of the month, a playful reference to a line from the Preamble.)

As you can see, AAs like to have fun with their group names and formats, and gay groups are no exception. But the names of the gay AA groups have always served a vital secondary purpose: to guide gay alcoholics to gay AA meetings without raising fear and alarm in the larger AA community.

Finding AA

Alcoholics Anonymous has no phone directory, no membership roster, and no mailing lists. Members find meetings by contacting their area's local AA service office, which maintains and publishes a local meeting schedule. Local schedules are also available at every AA meeting.

The first AA group directory, the predecessor of the current *AA World Directory,* was compiled in 1940 by the New York General Service Office (GSO). It was initially given to AA members who traveled in their work and were willing to visit people who'd written to New York asking for help starting an AA group. Starting in the 1950s, GSO began asking groups to send them a card containing their group name and the name and address of a member who was willing and able to receive GSO correspondence. This process became known as "registering" your AA group with the New York office. In turn, groups that had registered with GSO were listed in the group directory and received a copy of the *Group Secretary's Handbook and Directory.*

By 1953, GSO's directory listed 5,243 registered groups (Group Problems and Growing Pains 1953). Today, AA's *World Directory* consists of three volumes, each the size of a small phone book. There's one for groups in the eastern United States, one for groups in the western United States, and one for groups in Canada. A printed *International AA Directory* is also available, and a document called the *General Service Offices, Central Offices, Intergroups, and Answering Services Overseas* is now available on AA's Web site.

In the late 1960s, the secretaries of the first gay groups began writing to GSO and attempting to register their groups. They were often prompted to do this when their local AA office refused to include them in the local schedule. In New York, the GSO staff wasn't sure how to handle these requests. The general feeling at the time was that AA groups for homosexual alcoholics ought not to appear in the *World Directory*. But as the number of gay groups asking to be listed grew, the pressure to make a decision increased. Finally, in 1973, the GSO staff placed the issue before AA's annual General Service Conference.

But even after the gay groups began to appear in the *World Directory*, it was almost impossible to find them. Several factors contributed to this problem. First, not all of the groups in a given area register with the New York office. As a result, the *Directory* lists significantly fewer groups than actually exist. (For example, the *2002-2003 World Directory* lists 196 AA groups in San Francisco, but the locally published schedule lists nearly twice that number, 379.)

Second, the codes used in the local schedules to indicate the type of meeting listed (a "W" to indicate a women's group, for example) don't appear in the *World Directory*. So unless a group includes the word "Gay" or "Lesbian" in its name, readers cannot tell from the listing whether a meeting is for gay alcoholics or not.[1] And in the 1960s and early 1970s, stating openly in any publication that the members of your group were homosexuals was an enormous risk. Even today, very few gay AA groups include the words "Gay" or "Lesbian" in their names.

Finding AA in the Absence of a Press

Today, most of us are accustomed to seeing gay people portrayed in television shows and films, reading about gay organizations in the newspaper, and hearing gay people speak on radio or TV programs. So it can be difficult to imagine a time when homosexuality was completely absent from public discourse. Prior to the late 1970s, bringing up the subject was considered offensive, and people who viewed homosexuality as an illness were thought to hold a progressive point of view.

The concept of a "gay community," as we use and understand the term today, dates from the 1970s and the emergence of a gay press in the United States. Prior to that it was nearly impossible to share information with other gay people in your own city, much less with gay people in other cities or across the country.[2]

Until 1958, it was illegal to place printed materials containing the word "homosexual" in the U.S. mail (medical and religious texts being excepted). Materials that portrayed homosexuality in a positive light were classified by the government as "obscene." There were no gay books, or newspapers, or magazines. There were no bookstores to buy them in. It is hard to overstate how limited gay people were in their ability to communicate with one another prior to the presence of a gay press, and the profound isolation they experienced as a result.

Getting the Word Out

As gay AA groups formed in the late 1960s and began lobbying their local and national AA offices to include them in their directories, their members looked for alternative ways to publicize their meetings. The news traveled locally by word-of-mouth, and AA members who visited cities where they could attend a gay meeting brought home reports of their experience. In cities with an alternative newspaper, that is, one that would print the word "gay," AA members often placed an announcement that read, "Gay? Drinking problem? Call . . ." followed by the number of someone who could steer callers to a gay meeting. In the late 1960s, this notice appeared in Los Angeles in a news sheet called *The Advocate*. In San Francisco, the *Berkeley Barb,* a Bay Area weekly known for its radical views, carried the ad.

As word of the gay groups spread, new AA groups began to appear in more and more places. Starting in the 1970s, people like Nancy T., in Washington, DC, began compiling lists of the gay AA groups they knew about.

Not So Anonymous

In the 1960s, 1970s, and 1980s, gay AA groups and their members were subjected to surveillance, harassment, and other forms of intimidation by some of the more homophobic members of AA. Parking lots outside gay meetings were monitored to see who was coming out and going in. Gay members' automobiles were identified. Meetings were invaded in an attempt to shut them down. George M., who volunteered at the New York General Service Office for many years, reported hearing of a gay AA group in Australia whose members were told that unless they disbanded, their full names and addresses would appear in the local paper. Just how frequent and widespread such practices were is unknown, but it is clear that the members of gay groups were vulnerable to such attacks, and that they were afraid. Their sobriety, their jobs, their homes, families, and physical safety were at stake.

One of the strategies gay groups used to protect themselves was to place certain words, phrases, acronyms, and references in their group names that gay alcoholics would recognize, but straight alcoholics would not. This was also an effective way to get their meetings listed in local directories without indicating up front they were for gay alcoholics.

What's in a Name?

The most common name—by far—for an early gay AA group was "Live & Let Live," an AA slogan with special significance to AA's gay and lesbian members. Since many groups used AA slogans in their names, "Live & Let Live" drew no particular notice when it appeared in a local schedule. But to a gay AA member in search of a safe meeting, a Live & Let Live group was often a good place to start.

As the number of gay groups expanded, the words and phrases they employed in their names were adopted, modified, and reused by new gay groups. By studying old meeting schedules, I found that I could trace the growth of gay meetings in an area over time. In fact, I found groups meeting today that bear names directly related to gay meetings founded years ago in cities hundreds of miles away. For example, in 1979, adopting the practice of most AA groups in Milwaukee, Wisconsin, to use a number in their name, Wisconsin's first gay group became "Group 94." Subsequently, between 1979 and 1998, fourteen separate "94" groups appeared in Milwaukee, including Group 194, Group 294, Group 394, Group 494, and so on). In 1986, the "GB94" and "WB94" groups were founded in Green Bay and

West Bend, Wisconsin, respectively. And in 1988, the Fox River 94 Group was founded in Appleton, Wisconsin, and in 1990 the W94 Group was established in Waukesha, Wisconsin.

Here are some other creative AA group names that appear in Nancy T.'s early directories of gay and lesbian AA meetings:

- Freedoms Choice Group (Lafayette, Louisiana, 1983)
- Triangle Group (Washington, DC, 1998)
- Different Strokes Group (Sioux City, Iowa, 1983)
- A Different Light Group (Lawrence, Kansas, 1998)
- Drummer Group (Columbus, Ohio, 1979)
- Frankly Open Group (Atlanta, Georgia, 1979—with a nod to Rhett's famous parting line in *Gone with the Wind*).
- There's a Place for Us Group (Chester, Pennsylvania, 1998)
- Stepping Out Group (Danvers, Massachusetts, 1991)
- I Am What I Am Group (Baltimore, Maryland, 1998)
- We Are What We Are Group (Nashua, New Hampshire, 1991)
- Happy Campy Group (Sedona, Arizona, 1998)
- Open to All Group (Cambridge, Massachusetts, 1991)
- Oh, *That* Meeting! Group (Flint, Michigan, 1998)

Gay groups frequently employed acronyms in their names, dropping the intervening periods once the acronym became synonymous with "gay meeting." Chicago's first gay group was the GABS Group, short for "Gay Alcoholic Brothers and Sisters." Newer gay AA groups in the Chicago area adopted the acronym. For example, in 1986 in Geneva, Illinois, the Far West Suburban GAS Group, short for "Gay Alcoholic Sisters," was founded. Groups whose names included "GAA," short for "Gay AA," appeared in many locations across the United States. Other creative acronyms in the directories include:

- DT's Group ("Dykes Together," Atlanta, Georgia, 1979)
- GSG Group ("Growing Sober & Gay," Waterville, Maine, 1979)
- SAGA Group ("Sober and Gay Alcoholics," Wilmington, Delaware, 1982)
- GAYS Group ("Go After Your Sobriety," St. Petersburg, Florida, 1982)

- GALA Group ("Gay and Lesbian Alcoholics," St. Petersburg, Florida, 1998)
- GLASS Group ("Gay and Lesbian Alcoholics Seeking Sobriety," Portland, Maine, 1998)

Groups named "Alcoholics Together," as well as variations incorporating the words "Together" or "AT," were also common in the western United States after AT groups spread rapidly throughout southern California in the 1970s. San Jose's Men and Women Together Group and the PAT Group, short for "Peninsula Alcoholics Together," in Burlingame, a town on the San Francisco peninsula, are two examples. But only a handful of groups outside Southern California adopted AT's practice of requiring members to identify as both alcoholic and gay.

The word "Lambda" is still synonymous with "gay" in many parts of the world. Designer Tom Doerr used the symbol in 1969 in his logo for the Gay Activists Alliance, a political group that formed in New York City after Stonewall. References to famous gay and lesbian figures appear in the names of many gay AA meetings, including the Gertrude Stein Group in Santa Rosa, California, and the Oscar Wilde Group in Minneapolis, Minnesota.

My Quest for the First Gay Meeting

When I began studying the development of gay AA meetings, I had a great desire to find out which gay AA group had been The First. As a former San Francisco resident, I'd heard that our fair city was home to the first gay group. I must admit that I set out to prove this, and to bestow permanent bragging rights on my hometown. But, as is often the case, the more carefully I examined the data I'd collected, the more complex the picture became. Gay AA meetings were established in different ways at different times, under widely varying conditions. Just what, precisely, did it mean to be first?

Lesbians and gay men have been holding private AA meetings in their homes since the 1930s, when some of AA's first gay members got together in New York City. Were those the first gay AA meetings? In 1949 in Boston, a small group of gay men started a meeting in a local rooming house, though no evidence suggests that knowledge of this group extended beyond a small circle of trusted friends. Was this the first gay AA meeting?

In the 1950s and 1960s in New York, two primarily gay AA meetings met weekly in Greenwich Village, one nicknamed "The Saturday Night Follies," and the other, "The Red Door." These groups were listed in the New York AA directory, but not under those names, and not as gay meetings. (In this case, it was the groups' locations that indicated that gay people might be present.) Were these the first gay AA groups?

The first group to fit my modern definition of a gay group—the one most gay AA members would use today—was, in fact, the Friday Night Fell Street Group in San Francisco, established in early 1968. This group was

1. started by gay alcoholics, for gay alcoholics;
2. held in a public venue, rather than a private home; and
3. publicized as a gay meeting, inside and outside of AA.

The Fell Street Group was also one of the first gay groups to appear in the AA *World Directory* in 1975, and it was eventually listed in the local San Francisco directory as a gay meeting. The group continues to meet in its original location to this day.

So although I had failed to find the first gay AA meeting, I *had* ended up with a list of the conditions that often preceded the emergence of a gay AA group in a particular area. These include

- the presence of a local gay population, even a very loosely organized one;
- the presence of a few gay men or women who were established members of "regular" AA, even if they were very closeted;
- the presence of a local paper that would print the words "homosexual" or "gay"; and
- the presence of a church or other organization that would permit homosexuals to congregate on its property.[3]

Looking back on my search for the first gay AA meeting, I realized that, rather naively, I'd begun by looking for heroes—you know, those articulate, politically astute, spiritual visionaries who arrive in Alcoholics Anonymous. I imagined them on a rooftop somewhere, gazing steadfastly across the city skyline (their capes rippling in the breeze), proclaiming, "We shall start AA meetings for gay people! And we shall be free!"

Fortunately, the story is *way* more interesting than that. Besides, as far as bravery or spiritual bragging rights are concerned (and, God knows, we need more spiritual bragging rights), if awards are to be handed out they ought to go to the folks who started the first gay AA group in Memphis, Tennessee, or Des Moines, Iowa, or Salt Lake City, Utah.

So, I have abandoned my search for the first gay AA meeting. As far as I'm concerned, every gay AA group is the first gay group. Because regardless of when or where they began, each group had to establish itself within a larger heterosexual community, regardless of how large or small or dangerous or loving that community was. So please join me now in a toast to the first gay meeting of Alcoholics Anonymous, the one nearest the dessert table in heaven: the one in *your* neighborhood.

Chapter 6

Printer's Ink:
A Conversation with Nancy T.

In June 2002, I went to the Gay, Lesbian, Bisexual, and Transgender Historical Society in San Francisco to look around, and to see
if my idea for a book about gay people in Alcoholics Anonymous
(AA) might hold water. I spent the day there exploring, reading, and
talking with people. Late in the afternoon, a volunteer approached me
carrying a folder. "I just ran across this in our periodical files," she
said. "It might be relevant to your project." Indeed it was. She'd
handed me what turned out to be several issues of an old newsletter
published by the International Advisory Council of Homosexual
Men and Women in Alcoholics Anonymous, or IAC, for short. Inside
one of them was a brief account of IAC's founding, signed "Nancy
T____, Arlington, Virginia." Clearly, this was someone I should talk
to. But how?

After a discouraging evening of cold calling "Nancy T____s" in
the greater Washington, DC, area, I tried the numbers of the former
IAC chairs listed in the newsletter. Many of them had been discon-
nected, but I did eventually find someone who had an old telephone
number for Nancy. I gulped when she gave me the area code. "Did
you say, '415?' Good lord, that's San Francisco!" A few days later, I
reached Nancy and she agreed to meet with me. It was starting to look
like I had a real project on my hands.

The following Saturday, an atypically hot day in San Francisco,
I arrived on Nancy's doorstep for my first official project interview.
The house was an old Victorian in the city's Mission District. Think-
ing I ought to look official somehow, whatever an official lesbian

The History of Gay People in Alcoholics Anonymous
Published by The Haworth Press, Inc., 2007. All rights reserved.
doi:10.1300/5699_06

looks like, I'd donned business attire. I'd ditched my backpack for a briefcase and placed a notepad and a new tape recorder inside. Standing there in the heat I was still stunned that I'd found her at all, much less living nearby. I was nervous, excited, and overdressed.

Nancy came to the door wearing jeans and an Oxford shirt. She had dark brown hair, sparkling dark eyes, and I soon realized that I was in the presence of a Very Smart Person, albeit one with a practical, down-to-earth manner. She invited me into the living room and I sat on a small, Victorian-style sofa and tried to collect myself. The shades in the bay windows were drawn against the sun and heat. As my eyes adjusted to the light, I noticed many wonderful prints on the walls, some of which appeared to be by the same artist. Nancy went to get us some ice water. I began setting up my equipment, a fun activity that involved crawling around on the floor looking under furniture for an electrical outlet.

At last, the refreshments were ready, the tape recorder was ready, and Nancy settled into a chair across from me. I clipped the microphone to her collar and turned on the tape machine. But before I could say anything, she jumped up. Pulling off the microphone, she said, "Just a minute," and rushed out of the room. I heard her descending a flight of stairs. A few minutes later, she returned carrying a large, heavy file box that she dropped onto the coffee table with a thud. Reattaching the microphone, she began.

This box is entirely full of gay AA history. It has a variety of things in it and I'm going to turn it over to you. You can bring it back to me when we meet again. It contains a lot of things that will relate directly, or tangentially, to your project. *[Lifting the lid and pulling a folder out at random]* This is the list of people who were in IAC in 1991; this may help you find some of the old people. *[Pulling out another folder]* Here are old newsletters, old IAC directories, and an old IAC pin. *[And another]* This stuff relates to the history of the National Association of Lesbian and Gay Addiction Professionals [NALGAP]. These are early copies of what became the IAC directory and the NALGAP directory. It all ties in together. *[And another]* And here's what started it all: the pamphlet.

This is the pamphlet we thought would be published by the General Service Office. You'll find information in this folder [going]

back to 1982 when we began work on it. Here's the interview I did
with Dottie R. in 1991 before I moved to the Bay Area. Dottie was the
delegate from our area to the General Service Conference in 1981
and 1982. She is a progressive nongay woman who was very supportive of gay groups and very interested in AA history. You're welcome
to reorganize everything if you want.

I believe in turning stuff over and letting go. At one point, I turned
a lot of the early IAC-related materials I'd collected [over] to a member here in California and it disappeared. We have no idea what happened to it. Since then I've kept hold of every scrap, and I will track
you to your doorstep, and farther, if you lose hold of this.

I was a history major in college, and I have a strong appreciation
for history and for documents. I have carbon copies of just about all
my correspondence on all of these projects. I'm also a journalist.
[Laughing] I like to kid people and say printer's ink is my drug of
choice. So that's another reason that all this has been kept, and why I
drag it around with me.

Okay, so how all of these things happened, and how they fit
together—in other words, what does IAC have to do with the pamphlet, have to do with NALGAP, and have to do with the first gay
[AA] meeting in Washington, DC?

In 1969, I'd been a member of the Washington, DC, Mattachine
Society for about two years. Stonewall had happened, and Washington Mattachine decided they needed to do something. The Mattachine people knew I was a journalist and they invited me to be co-
editor of what we called the *Gay Blade,* now the *Washington Blade.* I
took over that project and eventually ended up as the sole editor. As
editor of the *Blade,* I went to a lot of different gay political meetings,
including meetings of Washington, DC's Gay Liberation Front,
where I met Bob and Cade, the two male cofounders of the Gay
Group of AA in Washington, DC. Bob and Cade subsequently introduced me to [cofounder] Blanche M. So I knew three of the four
founders of the first gay group long before I ever took my last drink.

At first, the Gay Group met in their homes, and when they wanted
to become public, they contacted me, as editor of *The Blade,* and they
asked me to publicize their meetings for them, which I did. I remember being very much in awe of them. The early 1970s was the
Women's Separatist Period of the Lesbian Movement—a time when

gay men and lesbians had very little to do with each other—and I was very impressed by the fact that these people were working together. And that they could stay away from drinking! I got sober in November of 1972; I was renting a room from Blanche when I went to my first AA meeting.

[During] my first year of sobriety, I learned that some people from the Washington, DC, group and some members of the gay AA group in Princeton, New Jersey, were working on a pamphlet for gay alcoholics. Cade knew I was in the publishing business and had experience working with small printers, so he and the others asked me to shepherd it into print. That is how the pamphlet *The Homosexual Alcoholic: AA's Message of Hope to Gay Men and Women* came into print. I had nothing to do with writing it, but I was its publisher, as such, and I subsequently felt a sense of responsibility to get copies to our group, to the Princeton group, and to other groups. I thought this was a very useful thing. This was early in the history of gay AA and people needed something that spoke to them.

At about this time [1974] I was beginning to travel in my business life, and whenever I traveled, I called ahead to the local AA office to find out if there was a gay group in the area, and there always was. I began to accumulate a list of these groups, and I sent them the pamphlet to see if they were interested in buying it, and they inevitably were. In the process, I accumulated information that led naturally to a list of gay groups around the country, which I then disbursed to the same groups. So the list fed off of the pamphlet, which fed off the list, and so forth.

So here we have the pamphlet and the list—the list of gay groups that led to associations with gay and lesbian alcoholism profession-als. I collected gay directories, like the *Gay Yellow Pages,* and some of these listed gay health clinics. When I discovered a clinic in a particular city, I'd call them up and they'd often direct me to AA meetings. It was a matter of calling around. People would say, "Oh, you ought to talk to so-and-so."

I put together a directory of gay and lesbian alcoholism resources that included papers on the topic published in the 1970s, a list of the clinics that hosted gay meetings, the names of alcoholism professionals who were themselves gay or lesbian that clients could be referred to, and the names of people studying alcoholism patterns in the gay and lesbian community, like they did in the clinics in Los Angeles.

So now we have three different resource sets: the pamphlet, the list, and the [professional] resource directory. The meeting list also included meetings of Alcoholics Together in Southern California, which were for gay alcoholics only. That's why the early versions of the listing were called *Meetings for Gay and Lesbian Alcoholics,* not *Gay AA Meetings.* Some people in Southern California were very adamant that straights be excluded from their meetings, and because they excluded straights, they could not be AA. The local AA hierarchy in Los Angeles did not want to list gay recovery meetings so everybody was at a standoff for a number of years.

Throughout the 1970s, I carried out most of this work pretty much solo. I was comfortable with it that way because I liked the control. Yet, on another level, I felt it was not a real AA effort because it was not a collaborative effort whatsoever.

In the process of creating and running all these lists, I had contact with people at the New York General Service Office [GSO]. I offered the GSO staff copies of *The Homosexual Alcoholic,* and they sent them to individuals and groups who inquired about the subject, even though it was not [AA General Service] Conference–approved literature. God bless them for doing that! In 1979 I offered the pamphlet to AA as a piece of hoped-to-be conference-approved literature, and they told me quite frankly that it would take years for that to happen.

We were approaching the 1980 International Conference in New Orleans, the first to have meetings for gay and lesbian alcoholics, and GSO asked me to help plan those meetings. I think we pulled together two great workshops, one with John W., the conference delegate from Washington, DC, who gave the history of the debates that occurred at the [1974] conference about admitting gay groups. At the other, we had a panel discussion led by gay people with long-term sobriety from different places in the country.

I was a good person for them to work with because I knew lots of people around the country, but I felt a profound sense of unease that I was the only person that they were working with on this. Even though the pamphlet had been written by gay people in AA, I had basically become the publisher over the years, and at that point, there was no institution to turn it over to. There was no IAC. There was no

NALGAP. And GSO had told me it would take up to five years for the piece to be reviewed—and reviewed and reviewed—by the General Service Conference.

Something needs to be in the world before then, I thought. If it's not GSO, what is the next most trustworthy institution to publish this? So at the 1980 International Convention in New Orleans, I went to see Hazelden at the hospitality suite they were hosting. Initially they were not terribly interested, until I told them I was selling 10,000 of them a year just on my own. That gave them pause! And in New Orleans I made arrangements to turn over the pamphlet copyright to Hazelden, knowing it was a way to get the message out to other gay and lesbian alcoholics beyond what I could do on my own. I sold the pamphlet to Hazelden for one dollar, and when I received their check a few months later, I put the dollar in the Seventh Tradition basket at the Gay Group and turned loose of it.

Washington, DC, had its second Roundup [gay AA conference] that August after the New Orleans conference. There was a big meeting—I don't remember the subject—and on the spur of the moment, I stood up and explained my dilemma.

"This should be a group project," I said. "I've been doing all this stuff over the years by myself. Does anybody else want to get involved?" Well, all kinds of people seemed interested! We began a correspondence—back then it was all by telephone and mail—and the following spring at the Boston Roundup [in 1981] we got together again, this time with people from different cities, and that was the beginning of what would eventually become IAC.

We argued about what to name the organization: "Lesbian and Gay Alcoholics" or "Gay and Lesbian Alcoholics"? What about the transgendered? What about this, and what about that? The only word we could compromise on was the most antique word, "Homosexual," and that's how it became the International Advisory Council of Homosexual Men and Women in Alcoholics Anonymous. We elected officers and I began divesting myself of my files. I was consulted a bit over the next year, and after that, I was out of it. As a courtesy, I compiled a couple more of the meeting directories for the group.

The third thing is NALGAP, and, again, it fits in. In the mid-1970s, Cade received a request [to speak] from the Rutgers Summer School of Alcohol Studies. Cade was never an AA sponsor of mine but he was a mentor, and he asked me if I'd be willing to work with him. I admired Cade tremendously. He had a great balance and dignity about him, and we worked well together. For three consecutive summers [1977-1979], Cade and I addressed the students of the Summer School as gay members of AA. Neither of us was an alcoholism professional; what we were was out-of-the-closet recovering alcoholics, and I didn't think I was really qualified to talk to them about gay and lesbian recovery.

By the third year, we had the wit to convene a meeting of gay and lesbian alcoholism professionals. Of course, all of them had been coming to our lectures. And once we did that, they wanted to become their own professional association. Dana F. and Emily M. became the first two copresidents. I was happy to turn over the materials I'd collected to them—the research papers, the information from people who'd corresponded with me who wanted information—and they, along with the other professionals, created this association.

Do you recall when you first started visiting gay groups on your business trips?

Probably 1974. By 1976 I was traveling a decent amount. I remember introducing myself to someone at a meeting in Dallas: "Hi, I'm Nancy T., from Washington, DC," and she looked at me and said, "Nancy T.? *The* Nancy T.?" And I had this awful sinking feeling. I'd always struggled not to let the ego stuff take over, and I knew this was a bad sign. It all always made me uneasy. Because first your ego gets out of control, then you risk drinking—drinking out of control. And I don't want people to see me for what my name is and not for who I really am.

What were some of the ways you found AA groups?

I combed the group directories published by the AA General Service Office, looking for names like the Lambda Group or the Live and Let Live Group. Back then, the group names were often coded. I would sit at the telephone at night and call these people around the country. I was also corresponding with people internationally to find out where groups were in other countries.

Did the local AA offices provide information about gay groups when you called?

The best reception I got was from Chicago. They were very friendly and outgoing. The worst reception I got was from Los Angeles. Somebody at the Los Angeles Intergroup office was very rude to me and rough when I called to ask for information about gay AA groups. It was a great contrast to what I got in Chicago, where people were very open.

Could you describe a typical conversation with a local contact once you found a gay group in a particular area?

They were usually very excited to know there were other groups forming around the country, and that I could send them the pamphlet and [gay meeting] lists. One night I ended up with somebody's ex-girl-friend on the phone. Her now-sober ex had moved out and left someone who was very angry. *[Laughing]* She practically hung up on me!

Temperamentally, the work suited me very well because I didn't have to interact with these people on a daily basis. They didn't see my daily frailties, my craziness, my psychic messes. They didn't have to deal with that person. They dealt with somebody in the far distance, and I dealt with them at a far distance, and it worked out very well.

Would you describe your publishing process?

I collected the information by making telephone calls around the country, corresponding with people, and meeting people at Round-ups. Then I'd sit down in front of the typewriter that fed information into our computer system, and when I got the type back, I proofread everything. In those days we ran the piece of paper through a waxer, did the prepress layout, and then I took it to a printer. That was the process used to publish the pamphlet and the various lists.

When I found people who were interested in the materials, I sent them out and placed the money they sent me into an account that I used to do the same thing over again, and again, and again. Whenever I published these things or corresponded with anyone, I always made sure to include a return address so people could send me more information.

I wanted a sheen of professionalism and distance there, and consistency, even though it was a part-time project. *[Laughing]* I was spending a lot of extra time at my office! There was a very permeable barrier between my professional life and my personal life. People urged me to find some official name for what I was doing but I never could. I had a real reticence to step forward. I called myself the project manager, although I never specified what the project was. It was just Nancy's project.

What were some of the publications you searched for listings?

Throughout the 1970s, I'd go down to the local gay bookstore and look through the newspapers. I'd find the calendars and get contact information from there. *[Laughing]* As I say, I was compulsive! But I was using my obsessions in a good fashion. An Al-Anon friend once told me that character defects and character assets are like reverse sides of the same sweater. There's a different pattern, depending on which side of the sweater you look on, but it's all the same fabric. I'm a collector. You can look around my house and see the various phases I go through—a particular artist, things from Japan, lesbian novels, postcards. In the twelve-year period we're talking about, I collected information. That was my collection.

So you picked up The Advocate *in Los Angeles?*

I read it in Washington, DC! The Lambda Rising Bookstore was the first gay bookstore in Washington, DC. I was friends with the man who founded it and he brought things in from all over so I was able to see things there. This was the first flowering of public gay life. We'd had Stonewall in 1969, and Stonewall begat a lot of organizations. Organizations begat bookstores, bookstores begat community centers, community centers begat newspapers, and newspapers begat books. I was surfing the crest of that wave, picking up what was of interest to me, which, at that point, was a very narrow spectrum of gay and lesbian life, the recovering alcoholic spectrum. That is a way I personally work very well—narrow spectrum, lots of depth.

So that's the timeline of it all, and you see why I needed to tell you, to refresh my memory. I put all those links together and, one by one, the pieces came off. Each time a responsible body was found to take over the work, I did whatever transitional tasks needed to be done, and then I walked away.

I'm proud that four things I've had a piece in creating—*The Blade, The Homosexual Alcoholic* pamphlet, IAC, and NALGAP—as far as I know, are all existing—all healthy, necessary things in the lives of people. If I had one thing carved in my headstone—if I had a headstone, which I'm not going to—it would be that I am the mother of those four things. *[Laughing]* I am happy that apparently I gave them a healthy enough childhood that they lived!

Chapter 7

Special Purpose Groups
and the Debate over Meetings
for Gay Alcoholics in AA

There was a lot of controversy about the presence of these few
little gay groups of AA within the fellowship. I was still pretty
new in April of 1974 when John W., our local delegate to the
General Service Conference, went to New York after coming to
our meetings many times that year. We were going to be debated
by those people, and I was so scared. I thought, *Schism. It's all
going to come now.* I remember turning to Cade after a meeting
when we were thinking, and praying, about the decision. "What
will we—what will I—do if they don't vote us in?"

Nancy T. (1986)
at the Fifteenth Anniversary of the Gay Group

Introduction

The debate over the inclusion of gay groups in the *World Directory*—AA's formal acknowledgment of its gay members at the national level—was framed by the discussion of "special purpose
groups." The issue of groups for gay alcoholics was first raised at the
General Service Conference in 1973. But meetings for particular
"kinds" of alcoholics had been around for years. For example, the author of "Fun with the *World Directory*," an article published in the
May 1963 issue of the *AA Grapevine,* noted that the 1963 *World Di-*

The History of Gay People in Alcoholics Anonymous
Published by The Haworth Press, Inc., 2007. All rights reserved.
doi:10.1300/5699_07

rectory listed 113 women's groups, fifty-eight men's groups, forty-seven young people's groups, and twelve different kinds of groups for AAs who shared a profession, such as those for doctors, policemen, pilots, and clergy.[1]

In AA, the term "special purpose group" generally denoted any group that wasn't a "regular" group of AA. These were typically groups whose membership differed in some way from AA's largely white, middle-aged, male majority. The following timeline gives a brief overview of the history of some of these groups.[2]

- The first AA group for women formed in Cleveland in 1941. By 1942, many of the women in New York AA (nearly forty at the time) were gathering regularly for a meeting of their own. By 1945, there were women's groups in Minneapolis and San Diego; Salt Lake City registered their first women's group with the General Service Office in 1952.
- The first AA group for black alcoholics met in Washington, DC, in 1945. The story of one of its cofounders appears in the book *Alcoholics Anonymous* ("Jim's Story"). By 1948, there were AA groups for black people in Missouri, Ohio, California, South Carolina, New York, New Jersey, and Pennsylvania. Twenty-five groups had registered with the General Service Office in New York by 1952.
- The first group for young people in AA convened in Philadelphia in 1946. Two years later there were "Thirty-Five and Under" groups in New York and San Diego, and it wasn't long before others were forming in cities around the country. The first International Conference of Young People in Alcoholics Anonymous (ICYPAA) was held in Niagara Falls, New York, in 1958.
- The first national AA convention for Spanish-speaking alcoholics in the United States was held in 1972. Today AA meetings in North America are conducted in many languages, including Spanish, French, Polish, Finnish, Italian, Korean, and Vietnamese. The first group for deaf and hearing-impaired alcoholics formed in Los Angeles. By 1982, GSO listed over 100 groups and AA contacts for deaf members.
- The first meeting of International Doctors in AA (IDAA) was held in 1949. There are currently several thousand AAs on IDAA's confidential mailing list. IDAA welcomes medical pro-

fessionals in a wide variety of fields, including physicians, surgeons, psychiatrists, psychologists, dentists, veterinarians, and research scientists.

- The first group for pilots in AA, originally called "Birds of a Feather," and now AA's International Pilots and Aviation Industry Professionals, met in Tacoma, Washington, in 1975. FAA regulations were such that pilots discovered to be alcoholic, even those with many years of sobriety, risked losing their jobs.

Today at many gatherings for AA members who share a profession, anonymity is still carefully guarded.

The Debate at the 1974 General Service Conference

In April 1974, AA members from across the United States and Canada gathered in New York City for AA's fourteenth annual General Service Conference (GSC). There, the twenty-one members on AA's General Service Board, including seven class A (nonalcoholic) and fourteen class B (alcoholic) trustees, the members of the General Service Office (GSO) staff, the *AA Grapevine* staff, and ninety-three elected conference delegates, met to discuss and vote on issues facing the organization as a whole. That year the conference turned its attention to an emerging controversy: Should groups for homosexual alcoholics be included in AA's *World Directory*?

Most of the arguments against listing gay AA groups centered on the feeling that they violated AA's Traditions. For example:

- Because the issue of civil rights for gay people was a controversial one outside of the organization, as well as inside AA, some held that listing gay groups violated AA's Tenth Tradition: "Alcoholics Anonymous has no opinion on outside issues; hence the AA name ought never be drawn into public controversy."
- Some felt that listing gay groups in the *World Directory* was an endorsement of homosexuality, and an endorsement of "gay rights," by Alcoholics Anonymous. This was seen as another violation of the Tenth Tradition.
- AA's First Tradition states, "Our common welfare should come first; personal recovery depends upon AA unity." Feelings on both sides of the issue were so strong that some pointed to the

controversy itself as evidence that gay groups were disrupting and dividing AA.

- Perhaps the most common argument against listing gay groups (and, by extension, the listing of any "special purpose" group) was that they appeared to exclude some alcoholics. Ironically, this was seen as a violation of the Third Tradition: "The only requirement for AA membership is the desire to stop drinking."

Old in AA, Big in AA, and Strong in AA

Another wonderful first-person account of the debate at the 1974 conference is preserved on a recording made at the workshop "Gays in AA: A Part of or Apart From?" held at the International AA Convention in New Orleans in 1980. The workshop's moderator, John W., was the 1974 delegate to the General Service Conference from Washington, DC. When the recording was made, John had also served as a Northeast regional trustee on the AA Service Board.

Following the talks given by the meeting's main speakers, John opened up the floor for discussion. A woman who'd traveled to the conference from Chile was the first to speak. A man from the audience named Eduardo volunteered to translate her remarks:

Hello, my name is Ruth. I am not gay, but I am an alcoholic. Like everyone here. I send greetings on behalf of the 5,000 Chilean AAs, to all of you. I have a very important question. The fellows of the group from Chile have a lot of trouble when they are gay, in order to go to the normal groups to preserve their sobriety. How can I, as a member of AA, as a member of Intergroup, help the great number of homosexual AA members in Chile?

At this point, Nancy T., who'd helped organize the workshop, addressed the assembly:

John, I think it would help Ruth, and Eduardo, and others here [from places] where there are no gay groups of AA, if you could give some of the history of the listing of gay groups in the *World Directory,* and about how an AA group qualifies for listing in the *World Directory,* and the relationship between gay groups and the local AA Intergroups. I think that's a fundamental problem in a lot of areas. People don't know how to get a group started, and how to get it listed.

"That's a big assignment!" John replied. When the laughter quieted down, he related the following.

Some years ago, when I was a delegate to the General Service Conference, there was a problem that was growing, and a feeling that was swelling up in certain parts of the country, about whether or not to list gay groups in our *World Directory*. The New York office wrote me a letter asking if I would make a presentation on this, and the heading this was going to be under was "Special Purpose Groups."

The real issue, I believe, was not special purpose groups, which means doctors' groups, stag groups, women's groups, lawyers' groups, gay groups, and so on. I think the real problem, and feeling, was gay groups, in some areas. Two of us, me and another delegate, made a presentation on this at the conference. [One spoke in favor, and one spoke against.] My presentation, to boil it down briefly, was that no matter who you are we should never shorten the hand of AA. No matter who you are. *[The audience cheers.]*

That April, we were supposed to decide whether or not to list special purpose groups. The presentations were on a Wednesday afternoon, followed by a two-hour discussion period, and it was some kind of fun. From the podium, you could tell that the feeling was split right down the middle—pro and con. But you could also tell that the real issue was the gay groups because most of the conversations had to do with "gay."

I don't know if any of you here have ever been delegates, but if you have not, in the conference meeting hall there is a center aisle and an aisle on each side. In those aisles are standing microphones, and after the presentations, if you wish to address remarks to the assembly, you stand behind a microphone. And pretty soon, it was like trying to get a ticket to the Super Bowl.

Two hours later they are beating the same damn drum. Fifty people over here are saying the same thing as fifty people over there. You could tell that the decision was not going to be reached; it was split down the middle. So we took a sense of the conference [a nonbinding show of hands to see how a vote might go] and decided that we would scrub the program for the following evening and go back into session on this subject and stay there, until it was finished.

Thursday evening it started again, just like a playback: the same lines at the microphones, the same things being said, over and over again, [and] nobody giving ground. Every once in a while, someone would say, "May I make a motion?" and the chairman would say, "No, not yet." When someone came to the mike, the chairman would ask, "Do you have a new point?" and [he or she would] say, "Yes." Well, the point was new Thursday night, but it was from Wednesday!

As the evening wore on—it was after ten o'clock, I think—you could sense that something was happening. Everybody, as it is in AA, had [had] a chance to get it off [his or her] chest. Then a delegate from Canada asked if he might make a motion. And the chair, sensing that it might be time, agreed. The motion was that gay groups be listed in the *World Directory,* and, right away, hands went up to amend the motion, to change it from "gay groups" to "special purpose groups," but the delegate would not change it. He said "gay groups" because that was the issue. "Do we, will we, recognize *gay* groups and list them in the *World Directory?*" The chairman called the question, and it was practically unanimous. And then, just as quick, a motion was made to amend it to include all special purpose groups.

It was quite a feeling, quite an experience, to see what we know as AA's group conscience at work, after everybody had spoken their prejudice, shall we say, after everybody had had their word. Believe me, it was quite a feeling, a very good one.

If you look in the *World Directory* you will see what an AA group is. It is simply two or three people gathered together for sobriety that have no affiliation with any outside causes, that are self-supporting, and so on. It's just that simple. It doesn't say, "Are you white? Are you black? Are you gay? Are you straight? Are you wealthy? Are you on relief? What language do you speak?" It says that you are bound together to help one another because you are ill, and that your primary purpose is to stretch out your hand. This is what AA is all about. *[The audience cheers.]*

[When the applause has subsided, John continues.] Speaking of Intergroups, you say there are problems in some areas? Well, you'd better infiltrate them. *[There's a burst of laughter and cheering.]*

Let me qualify that. *[More laughter]* Let me tell you a story from my experience, and I think you will understand what I'm saying.

I am from Washington DC. Originally, I'm from Ohio, but I've been in Washington for a long, long time. I got sober there and became very active in the fellowship. Washington, DC, as you know, is predominantly black, and when I became Intergroup chairman, there was not one black person on the Intergroup desk.[3]

Now, Washington is old in AA, it is big in AA, and it is strong in AA—black and white. The first black group in AA history started there, and it's still operating. Dr. Jim, one of the original stories in your Big Book, was a colored doctor from Washington. And yet, as active as black AAs were, there were no black people on the Intergroup desk, or on the Intergroup committee, and one of my secret things that I was going to do was to crack this. Only because I thought it was basically un-AA and wrong. Also, at the time I came in, the black AAs weren't too welcome at most of the other groups, and I stuck my nose in that too.

I talked to some of the good, old-time black members—one man, and one woman, especially, who were beautiful people. I told them I needed their support because I was going to try to get black workers on the desk. It was so silly. At our monthly Intergroup meetings, there were problems: [e.g.,] "The desk workers are having trouble. What should we do?"

One of the problems was, "When somebody calls and you've got them on the phone, how do you tell whether they're black or white? You can't always tell by their accent."

Another was, "How do you know whether to get a black person or white person? You can't even tell by the address anymore."

So I made it known at the Intergroup committee meeting that I thought it was time we did this, that I'd be happy to stick my neck out, that I'd take full responsibility, and I got them to agree. Then I went back to my two friends.

"We are going to have black people working on the desk, and black groups are going to have representation, but I need your help. I can't do it alone. You must select from among you those people who are big enough, and strong enough, and sober enough to take what they might have to take, from time to time, from certain people—the prejudice. They will have to be bigger."

That's what I mean by infiltrating a little bit. It's like anything else. If you have this problem in your area, talk to someone who has been or is interested or active at Intergroup, who you know is AA all the way, up and down. If you know what I mean by that. Ask them to help you, and you can work it out.

In the beginning, some of the black people had to—Nobody was nasty, but there was a coolness. You know what I'm going to say. There was that feeling. But it worked out. I went a little too fast on it and had to back off. Once the first thing worked I wanted to do something else in a hurry, and I got kicked in the shins for that. But nonetheless, it has worked out beautifully. And I think the same can be true with gays, or anyone else.

Thank you.

*   *   *

In 1974, in formal recognition of gay people's presence and full membership in Alcoholics Anonymous, the members of AA's General Service Conference voted almost unanimously—128 to 2—to list gay groups.

Today, a very similar debate absorbs Americans—in churches, temples, synagogues, and schools; in state and federal congresses and assemblies; in our courts: Are gay people entitled to full membership in our society?

PART II:
BUILDING SOBER COMMUNITIES,
1970-2004

In the narratives that follow, men and women who came into Alcoholics Anonymous between 1961 and 1981 in different parts of the United States share their stories. Some were in AA long before the gay groups started. Others found gay meetings waiting for them in AA and encountered knowledgeable staff at hospitals, social service agencies, and treatment centers. You'll also hear from more pioneering professionals whose work has changed the way the world thinks about addiction and about gay alcoholics.

Chapter 8

Washington DC

Blanche M.

[Blanche got sober in Washington DC, in 1969. She is a cofounder of the first gay group of Alcoholics Anonymous (AA) in Washington, DC.]

In 1966, I couldn't admit or even know I was an alcoholic, but I was terribly disturbed by how emotionally ill I was. I was living in Washington DC, and had recently gotten married. I was a housewife and a daily drunk.

When I got married, I'd left a relationship with a woman. Lynn and I were stewardesses in the 1950s and had been for many years. Word got out that we were gay, and I was asked to leave the airline. Lynn continued to fly. We moved to New York. We didn't acknowledge between the two of us that we were gay. We had no gay friends. We were totally isolated and locked within one another. Lynn went into nursing school, and I helped her through that. She started to become more mature in the relationship, and to find other friends.

My husband-to-be [Cal] kept coming up to New York. He had a lot of money, and we'd go to the best places. He wanted me to take a three-carat [diamond] ring. I saw Lynn starting to get a life of her own, and I was in anguish over what to do. Cal . . . wanted me to buy a Jaguar convertible, and I gave in to that—that and the pressure of my family, and society. . . .

One day we were sitting in Cal's apartment [in Washington DC]. I was drunk and he was drunk, and on the spur of the moment, he called

The History of Gay People in Alcoholics Anonymous
Published by The Haworth Press, Inc., 2007. All rights reserved.
doi:10.1300/5699_08

up a minister and off we went. He wanted me to be a housewife, which was pretty much the thing to do back then. *Great,* I thought *Why not?* I had my own little Porsche. We had a beautiful home, and we had a cabin cruiser [yacht]. But I went from a person who drank heavily on weekends, to a person who just sat home, day in and day out, and drank.

I could not face the fact that I'd left Lynn. In my drunken state, I would call her and beg her to come live with me. I'd drive up to Long Island to visit her and couldn't get sober enough to come back. I put her through agony.

I was under a psychiatrist's help. Back then, you lay on a couch, and you would not see him. If you talked, there would be no interaction. I would talk about the anguish of leaving Lynn. I'd say, "I really am gay. I don't know why I have married." But he was back in the Freudian days where, if you didn't have a climax in the vagina, you were still immature. That's the kind of professional help you had back then.

I went to Washington Hospital Center to come off of a particularly bad drunk. Most of the people in the ward weren't alcoholics. They were in for severe mental problems. I kept walking around my room. The night nurse saw me and said, "Come on out in the hall. We'll walk up and down together." She dragged two chairs, dragged them all the way down to the end of the floor, and we sat.

"Do you think," I asked her, "now that I've been in here, that I won't be drinking anymore?"

"Well, that's going to be up to you. You may want to look at the fact that you are an alcoholic."

I was so humiliated. I'd come from a very nice upbringing, and to me, drunks were just the dregs! I couldn't see myself being one of them.

"An alcoholic? I just get very sick when I drink."

"You asked me, 'Do you think I'll ever drink again since I've had to be in here?' That answer is going to have to come from you."

When I got out of there I started going to meetings. I sat in the corner of the room and hardly said anything, and I was squirrelly with withdrawals. My social phobias were unbelievable. I recognized that I had no hope. We've heard this before. I was at that place where I didn't want to die, and I didn't want to live.

From March to August, I was in and out, in and out, but I did meet two wonderful women. "Blanche," [they said,] "why don't you give the program six months? If you still feel like committing suicide [then], then go! But give yourself six months. See if you don't feel differently." And of course, it was happening. I was watching people get better, seeing them laugh, and making friends.

The last time I went to see Lynn I'd been drunk every day. Now it was time to leave and I was too sick to come home. She didn't think I should drive. She wanted me to come in and lay down with her. "If I do, I'll never go back," I said, and I had my last drink of alcohol on August 30, 1969.

By the fall of 1971, I knew I was definitely gay. Once in a while, I'd go to the Capitol Street meeting, and I don't recall whether I'd seen Cade or Bob there before, but one night I noticed that Cade was wearing a button [on his lapel that said], "Gay is good." I kept looking at that button. *He must be crazy, wearing a thing like that,* I thought. I kept looking at Cade, and looking at Bob. I didn't know what gay guys looked like!

After the meeting, I went over to Cade and tapped the button. "Is this for real?"

"Yes, it is," he said, "and I'm very proud of it."

We went [that night] to Mr. Henry's coffee shop on Capitol Hill, and I talked and talked about being gay, and they were so helpful. I knew no other gay people, and they gave me the names of two gay women and organizations in town that I could call. They also told me about a woman [in AA] named Gerry Kay who was still drinking.

She had been calling them about a difficult breakup she was going through. "It's so hard going to straight meetings," she'd say, "where I've got to pretend my relationship is with a man. I wish we could get together to discuss our alcoholism and our sexuality."

We went to Mr. Henry's again, and talked about getting a group together, and then we did some soul searching.

What exactly are my motivations for doing this? I wondered. *I got sober in straight AA. Has it failed me? What would I say to my sponsor?* I didn't know of any other group that had done this, and what kind of group would it be? I wondered if I was trying to get attention in some sick way. Bob and Cade were feeling many of the same things, though I think they felt the time had come. They were much more courageous about going forward than I was, but, then, they had their friends. . . .

I was [still very closeted and very] uncomfortable. What if this gets out? [Meanwhile,] Gerry Kay, who was still out there drinking, was always in the background, saying, "Let's go for it."

One night I found myself just blurting everything out during one of those talks with Cade and Bob. Up until then I had never had a chance to explain my drinking, how connected it was to leaving Lynn, how much I'd wanted to talk about the anguish of leaving her, and never could. I spilled everything out, and they listened. Driving home that night, I felt such relief. *My god. I feel so good. If this is happening to me, are there other people who might feel this way?* We knew Gerry Kay was, because she kept calling us. She would be drunk quite a bit of the time, but her message was clear.

My sponsor was the last person I talked to [about the meeting], and she should have been the first. When I told her what we were thinking about, she looked at me and said, "I think it's a wonderful idea. Wonderful."

It was early fall in 1971 when we brought Gerry Kay in, and then we had the four of us. The meeting was at Cade and Bob's [house] on Capitol Hill one week, and at my house in Alexandria the next. My husband and I had split, and I was staying in our house until it sold. I used to look down the hill and see them walking up my driveway, and my feeling was, *Oh my god. I hope the neighbors don't see this.* By this time I was starting to recognize people who might be gay, and about the next Sunday, Tom H. came walking up the steep driveway, and my feeling was, *Get in the house! Get in the house, before anybody sees you! Because you look too gay to me!*

I was very closety and not at all comfortable about the direction my sexuality was taking me. There were a few of us early on, I found out, who felt like me—scared to death to go to a meeting in case we were seen. I didn't know whether I wanted to be around a bunch of gay people. I was so embarrassed. What if I were to be found out?

Now there were seven of us: me, Bob, Cade, Gerry Kay, then Barbara and Andrea, and then dear old Tom, coming up the hill. We wondered if we could find a church that would allow us to hold our meetings there. We thought, *Oh, this is going to be good.* [First] we tried the Capitol Hill area. Then we approached another church further out, and Cade and Bob called to say we'd been turned down again. Then they tried St. James Episcopal Church. The priest's lover had been an alcoholic, and he welcomed us with open arms.

Bob had written to a gay alcoholics' group in Los Angeles and told them we were thinking of starting a gay group and asked if they had any advice. A letter came back saying, "Forget it! It's going to turn out to be one big, fat, happy social hour, and nobody's going to stay sober." The message was that it was going to be nothing but a pick-up place, and that there were no women, which reinforced what I was thinking: *This is going to be a bunch of gay, in-your-face guys.*

Most of the people in the group were men. . . . It was rocky for me, and for Barbara, before she left. I felt put down and overwhelmed by the laughter, and the talk about who they went out with the night before, and who they were going to have sex with that night. They were overtaking the meeting and there was little I could say. I wanted to talk about some things along the lines of women, and they didn't want to hear any thing about it. There were two guys in particular who obviously didn't care for women, and they caused concern in our early meetings.

Then Ellen joined the scene, and she was a bit more like me. One night, Ellen and I drove to the meeting together, and as we walked toward the building, we saw a fire burning near the church. A few moments later, the fire engines arrived, and Ellen, who had a big professional job, thought the church was being raided because we were a gay group, and she ran up the alley. I ran after her, calling, "No! Ellen, no! Don't worry! It's just a fire!"

That's how we were feeling back then. But we kept going, and I hoped things would eventually balance out. It took a few months for everybody to settle down and really start having an AA meeting, but that's exactly what happened.

Then a women's meeting started. At the gay women's meetings, we felt comfortable with one another. There we could talk *our* talk. When I got with a bunch of gay gals, we got into serious talk about how worthless we felt, which is pretty common, whether you're gay or straight. I seldom hear guys talk about worthlessness, or low self-esteem. We talked about self-esteem, about having to leave husbands, about coming out later in life, about still being mixed up as to whether we were truly gay or not, and about our guilt for having been gay.

When I see this younger generation, just so open with themselves, and so at home with it, I think, *God, I wish—* I don't wish that things had been different for me. My challenges have been interesting, if painful. But everybody's come so far, so far! I came from a well-to-do family. "What will the neighbors say?" was my background. You go to college, you get married, you become a housewife, and then, if you have this other side of your nature, screaming—

To be comfortable with being gay took me many years. But once in a while, I say to my Higher Power, *Well, if I was to be gay, at least I was in on this very important thing that turned out to be so needed:* [the founding of the gay group].

When we got more people in the gay group there was no more reason for me to spill everything out. Cade had had his time, Bob had had his time, and I'd had my time. By then, other people were coming in and going through the catharsis we had gone through. Time and time again, we'd start the meeting and, all of a sudden, it would be Tom. He'd talk for an hour; you could see the tears in his eyes. You could see the relief in his face. *That's* what I look back on and feel so good about. I often think of it because I was such a doubting Thomas about my life and my sexuality. I feel humbled by how far it's all come.

I've sponsored many people in my later years. My straight sponsor breathed life into me, and loved me. Marilyn and Karin guided me well, and I got a thorough grounding from them on how to sponsor when it came my time. When I got a certain amount of time [in AA], I saw that I'd gone through many crises and that somehow I got through [each one]. You don't drink, and you learn, and I continue to learn. I'm willing now to talk a little at a straight meeting about my conflict with being gay. Afterward people will come talk with me, or a month later I'll have a phone call, out here in the country, especially. I'm active in a little AA clubhouse we got up and running a few years ago. Not many people here sponsor anyone, and if they do, they've never had a sponsor to [teach them] how to sponsor. I'm sponsoring about twelve people right now, and each person is different. It keeps me honest. I can't sponsor anybody unless I continue to do what I'm suggesting that they do!

There's no other way to say it. I owe my life to AA, and AA is still a very exciting experience to be involved in. I'm in my late sixties now. I see how precious life is before me, and how my struggles have made me more compassionate. I still work on my character defects. I've come to understand what it means to forgive and not look to be forgiven, to give love and not look for anything back. The St. Francis of Assisi prayer says, "Where there was darkness, now there is light." I see that at meetings. People come in so sick [and] then they get better.

David C.

[David got sober in 1974 in Washington DC. I spoke with him where he works, at the AA Service Center in Contra Costa County, California, east of San Francisco.]

At twenty-eight I was at the end of my path. For three nights in a row, I'd gone to the roof of the building where I lived, to jump off, and each night I'd change my mind. On the fourth night, I came out of a blackout on the ledge of the building, with my legs hanging over the side, fourteen stories above the parking lot.

The next morning I called AA. I told the woman who answered the phone I wanted some information for a friend. She asked me how old my friend was and I said I was twenty-eight, that we were both twenty-eight, and she suggested that we might want to go to a young people's meeting. She said it would be wonderful support for us and that the Thursday Night Young People's Group met that evening on Woodley Place.

That night I raced home from work [and] changed into the grungiest clothes I could find. I was afraid that if I showed up wearing a business suit at an AA meeting—in a cellar, with a bunch of drunks—that I might never see the light of day. Then I ran back to Dupont Circle, up Connecticut Avenue to Woodley Place, and into the cellar of this church, past a room full of clean, happy-looking people. Sunday school teachers or something. But the further down the hall I got, the darker [the hallway became].

When I turned around, there was a young man standing by the door of the room I'd passed.

"Can I help you?"

"No thanks. I think I'm in the wrong place."

"Don't be so sure. Are you looking for Alcoholics Anonymous?"

"Why, as a matter of fact, I—"

"I'm Michael," he said, putting out his hand. "I'm an alcoholic."

Michael was about nineteen, an all-American poster boy for recovery. I believe he was an angel placed there to greet me at my first meeting.

I became a member of the gay groups, and I went to the others as well, so I blended. I never stayed within the gay groups only, and I'm grateful for that, but I see the importance of a safe harbor.

When I got sober, Cade W. and Bob W. were already AA members and we renewed our friendship. I first met them through the Gay Activists Alliance [GAA; in Washington DC]. I'd been to some GAA meetings but hadn't joined because, if you weren't available to be out and proud, they didn't need you. They didn't need an auxiliary of closeted members.

The first GAA activity I was involved in came in response to an incident at a dinner and dance club on Connecticut Avenue. One evening a gay couple danced together, and they were told to get off the dance floor. When they refused, the management turned on the bright lights, told the orchestra to stop playing, and instructed everyone to leave the building. That was a turning point for me. I felt that if I didn't become involved in it then, I was going to end up being pushed, farther and farther, into the alley. When the Gay Activists Alliance picketed this restaurant, I was part of it.

In 1975, I started to think about moving to California. A man I'd met in AA had moved to California, and for my thirtieth birthday, I went to visit him. The moment I saw San Francisco, I knew I could no. longer live in Washington DC. Earl was a charming fellow and I took to him like an old friend. We had a long platonic relationship until he died in 1981. I also visited Long Beach [on that trip], where I attended my first Alcoholics Together [AT] meeting, where you were required to identify yourself as both an alcoholic and a homosexual before the meeting, or you were asked to leave. I found this rather retrogressive, but I'd been part of mainstream AA in Washington DC, and had had the advantage of many straight supporters, so I figured there must be some particular need for this in Southern California.

In 1975, there were four gay meetings in San Francisco: two at the Congregational church on Post at Mason, Friday night on Fell Street, and a wonderful noontime meeting at Hospitality House, on Leaven-worth. *[Laughing]* It was a dreadful little place. I was the coffee maker [there for] awhile, and we were always collecting tin cans to keep the rats out of our supplies.

I understand you were involved in planning the first Living Sober conference in 1976. How did it get started?

My understanding is that the idea came out of some people's experience at the gay hospitality suite at the 1975 international conference in Denver. There were movers and shakers who did most of the organizing. I was one of the few with a full-time job, so I did things like buy postage stamps and paper. *[David becomes quiet.]* I'm starting to get emotional, thinking of so many of us who are no longer here.

I was the secretary for the nighttime meeting marathon that first year. Other than the guard, I can't remember anyone coming in, but I do remember going to Fisherman's Wharf and buying a plaid carrying case with thermoses and a sandwich box inside. I baked cookies and took coffee for the meeting overnight.

After the conference the number of gay AA groups seemed to proliferate. I think getting the word out—I'm not saying we broke AA Traditions when we spread the word, but we were out. We were out, and we were proud! . . . Many of us had experience as members of the Gay Activist Alliance and, earlier, the Mattachine Society. The first Living Sober did not attract a lot of long-term AA members in the community. It broke with tradition [to be so open], and, perhaps, given the character of some of the people on the planning committee, it appeared too extreme. But it didn't take long before these people were attracted to Living Sober. Within a year or two, they joined the tribe, and, in doing so, strengthened it.

Later, at the twenty-fifth Living Sober conference, "we were termed pioneers." We didn't think of ourselves as pioneers. I mean, for heaven's sake, in 1976 we weren't sure we'd make it to the conference, much less the next year or ten years down the road. To me, that first gathering was a testimony to freedom, that we would not be restricted from meeting and carrying our message, and our experience [to the alcoholic who still suffers] for lack of a venue.

How did you come to Contra Costa County, and to the AA Service Center?

I've had four partners in recovery, and *[smiling]* of course, my dream was that some young fellow would allow me to retire early, and keep me the way I was accustomed. But that has not been the case. All four lovers have gone by the epidemic. For some reason, I am still here. My last partner passed away twelve years ago yesterday. *[He grows quiet.]*

Austin and I decided we wanted to experience the gay, clean, and sober American dream. In 1986 we left the Castro and bought a home in Concord [a small town in Contra Costa County], our own piece of suburbia. When we arrived, there was a homophobic preacher here named Lloyd Mayshore, whose goal was to remove all public servants from their posts, if they could be proven to be gay. But we came prepared to survive. We weren't going anywhere. We weren't demonstrative in public; they were looking for us. The first couple of years we had no more than four or five confrontations with people who were very angry at having a gay couple in the neighborhood. But we weathered those storms. We had it all: the house, the pickup truck, and our two golden retrievers, Sam and Meg.

Six months later Austin was diagnosed with AIDS, or HIV; we thought there was a difference at the time. He lived for two and a half years, and we got to enjoy our dream together. One of his last comments was that we should write a book called *Fast Forward* because we'd lived an entire lifetime together in a few short years. *[David's eyes fill with tears, and he weeps.]* Austin died sober, in 1990.

My commitment to Austin was that I'd keep the house here as long as the kids needed the yard. When Sam died, I got Serene to keep Meg company, and when Meg died last year, I adopted Pacheco to keep Serene company. *[Laughing]* So my commitment was to stay as long as the kids needed the yard, but I probably won't outlive the kids I've since acquired! Chances are.

Now the gay AA groups out here have increased. One has started right here at the Service Center. A new meeting called the Freedom Rings Group is also growing. [It has] a delightful mix of gay, lesbian, and straight members. I believe an incredible mingling of gay and straight people is taking place in AA.

I was in a men's meeting recently, at the Alano Club in Martinez, with a friend who also got sober in 1974, a gruff, motorcycle type. Don had been with the mob, in their retribution program in New York and [Las] Vegas. He knew me with no secrets and respected me as an individual, and a friend. He knew Austin too, and that Austin had died. Don chaired the meeting [was the speaker that night], and at one point he said that it was in that men's meeting that he'd [first] realized he could hug another man and not be considered a faggot. When he was through speaking, I raised my hand. I thanked him for his story, and for the lesson he had just taught me.

"There happen to be faggots in this room," I said, "and I think you can never really tell when there will be or won't be. And if there's someone here tonight who happens to be a faggot, particularly if you're new, please feel that this home is yours. Don't let the message you hear here drive you into death, away from these rooms."

Then Don apologized profusely, not only to me but to the group for his lack of judgment, and that opened doors for that group. It opened up the topic for people who would not normally talk about it, and I think a seed was carried out of that room.

I have not had a partner since Austin died, and that has enabled me to be of service to Alcoholics Anonymous. One of my great joys has been working with other men in recovery. I've had many more straight sponsees than gay sponsees, and I find that completely compatible with staying sober and working with others. Bob K. has been a great inspiration to me.[1] In his first meeting he was three sheets to the wind! Bob has been active and available to other gays and lesbians in Contra Costa County and has also been very representative in the mainstream of AA.

Each of us has had trailblazers on whatever path we're on. Cade W. taught me it was all right to be a mainline educated citizen, out and proud. Nancy T. and her lover Loren were the first lesbians I ever knew. Loren started the gay Al-Anon meetings on Capitol Hill. Ed B. and John C. were very successful in the business world, and very closeted, but they wouldn't miss a meeting. Another dear friend who's died recently was Eileish L., who founded First Place, the gay AA meetinghouse on Post Street in San Francisco. Eileish was one of the straight saints among us.

There were people there to open the door for me when I arrived, and now I'm holding the door for people who might be less secure. There's a young man who comes to meetings at the Service Center. He's an incredibly effeminate young person, and still in search of himself, obviously, at that age. He knows that I am gay, that I'm in the mainstream, and that he can talk to me. What an opportunity it is to hold the door open for others who follow us in life!

There's a one-liner that goes around the rooms of [AA]: "Whoever got up earliest this morning has the most sobriety." Well, that's very cute, but it doesn't make sense if I believe that recovery is progressive. Surely, if [you have] traveled this path a long time, [you] have developed a gift [you] could not have had a day sooner.

Chapter 9

New York

George M.

[George got sober in New York.]

In 1974 my partner and I owned a house in Cherry Grove on Fire Island. I spent three summers out there, ostensibly using the peace and quiet to do some writing, but it became a no-holds-barred, summer-long drinking binge. It was a great place for an alcoholic. There being no cars, you couldn't become involved in a drunk-driving incident, or walk in front of one. And if you fell down a lot, as happened to me, most of the time you fell on sand. Or possibly poison ivy.

The final year I was out there a neighbor kept an eye on me. I knew he'd stopped drinking, so I avoided him. Worse yet, he actually talked about it. . . . It was bad enough if you were one of those unfortunate people who couldn't drink, but to bring it up in polite company seemed beyond the pale. He grabbed me on a day I felt so ill I would have talked to the devil himself, and persuaded me to go into the Central Islip State Hospital detox. I didn't fully understand what that meant, but the notion of being in the hospital made sense, and I was trucked off to the locked detox ward.

When I returned to New York City, I called a woman I knew had joined AA, and abandoned the rest of us and asked if she still went to those meetings. [She said,] "Oh yes, honey. I do." and she took me to meetings in Greenwich Village for a week.

I wanted to know everything about AA. I wanted to know everybody who was important—all the stars, the VIPs, the power brokers. *[Laughing]* It took me a while to realize that wasn't so likely.

The History of Gay People in Alcoholics Anonymous
Published by The Haworth Press, Inc., 2007. All rights reserved.
doi:10.1300/5699_09

For all intents and purposes, the meetings I went to were exclusively gay. The one exception was the Perry Street Workshop Group, which is something of a legend in New York AA. It was the second group to form in Manhattan, splitting off from the first one in the early 1940s because they didn't like all the God talk. To this day, they rent what at one time was a Chinese laundry on Perry Street in the Village.

The Workshop didn't put a lot of pressure on new members about believing in God. This was great for me because at the point I joined AA I was a militant, outspoken atheist, and the one thing I could not tolerate was anyone who wasn't just as open-minded on the subject. . . .

In January of 1975, the AA Intergroup office got an appeal from the National Council on Alcoholism [NCA] for volunteer help and I quickly became involved in a number of things they needed help with. They found a clerical position for me on staff and I remained there for fifteen years. When I told Marty I'd ended my drinking in Cherry Grove, it turned out she'd spent time there and knew some of the same people I did. We never had any in-depth conversations about gay things. She told me, as she told some other people she encountered along the way, that she didn't make an effort to conceal that she was gay, that in order to educate people about alcoholism as a treatable disease, she felt it was important not to add any other stigma or confusing issues.

For a long time I didn't really see a connection between being gay and being alcoholic, and I'm careful about suggesting there could be a cause-and-effect relationship between the two. I don't know of any evidence that there is, and it can be very stigmatizing to suggest that being gay makes you alcoholic, or vice versa. [However,] I do think gay people are much more at risk for alcoholism, for a whole bunch of reasons, beginning with homophobia, heterosexism, and the stress [that] those create. Stress is an identifying risk factor for substance abuse. People who are under constant stress are more inclined to turn to alcohol and drugs. Gay communities are also heavily targeted by alcohol and tobacco companies. . . .

In 1976, *The Advocate* [a Los Angeles news sheet, at the time] published a series of articles on alcoholism in the gay community, written by Randy Shilts, whose name meant nothing to me at the time. I clipped those articles and saved them.[1] Later, when the National Association of Lesbian and Gay Addiction Professionals [NALGAP] was established, [NALGAP cofounders Dana Finnegan and Emily McNally] made contact with me at NCA, and Natalie Becker—a brilliant woman who was neither gay nor alcoholic, who I then reported to—said, "Why don't you organize a track on [alcoholism in the gay community] for the 1980 National Alcoholism Forum?"

The National Alcoholism Forum was NCA's annual conference and the largest conference on alcoholism in the country at the time. So with the help of [Dana and Emily], and a couple of other people, we planned a [conference] track on gay alcoholism.

I dredged those [*Advocate*] articles out of my file, and saw that the information Randy had used was based on an unpublished study done by Lillene Fifield, in Los Angeles. I don't know what prompted them to fund it in the first place, but the state of California and the Los Angeles County Department of Health gave [Lillene] a little bit of money and no time at all to find out about alcoholism among gays in Los Angeles. She did her study and wrote up the report, which was never released or published at all. A short synopsis version did get printed two or three years later. It got very minimal distribution, and that was it.

I tracked Lillene down in Roseburg, Oregon, where she was living, and asked her to come to the conference and be the keynote speaker. She was absolutely dumbfounded, because from the moment she'd typed her report on her survey in Los Angeles County, nobody, except Randy Shilts, had ever wanted to hear about it.

"No one has ever wanted me to talk about this," she said, "and now, you're asking me to come to Seattle?"

"Can you?"

I asked and she said that she would.

At the time, her study and two other small studies were all that had ever been done to quantify the problem in our community, and we were all very excited about it, because the studies had all come in saying that about 30 to 33 percent of the respondents showed signs of alcoholism which made the case that we deserved resources and services. But all this backfired on us very quickly because none of us who ran with this information were researchers, and [we didn't understand] what we were looking at.

Lillene had done her survey primarily among regular patrons of gay bars in Los Angeles County, and the other two had been samples mainly of people in jails and institutions. And anytime you look at those populations, whether they're gay or straight, you're going to see very high levels of alcohol consumption. And with high levels you'll see indicators of possible alcoholism, but that's not to say you are seeing alcoholics. So academics began attacking this research pretty quickly, and later it began to occur to some of us that it reinforced negative stereotypes of gay people, and created terrible expectations for kids who were coming out.

However, if you go back and read Lillene's study, as I have done, you will see that she never said that a third of the community was alcoholic. She said that a third of the community was alcoholic or showed signs of possibly developing alcoholism, which is true, and is still true now. But you need to understand drinking patterns to interpret that correctly.

Showing signs of possibly developing alcoholism doesn't necessarily mean anybody ever will. In young male drinkers in the United States, you see about 30 percent in their twenties who would meet the criteria for alcoholism treatment, but when you look at the same group ten years later, about two-thirds of them have fallen out, and what remains are the people who have alcoholism or alcohol dependency. As most people reach age thirty, their alcohol consumption begins to decline, often spontaneously, without their giving it any thought it all.

I am trying to learn more about Barry L. Did you ever encounter him at meetings in New York City?

I knew Barry, and took to him quickly. He made no bones about the fact that he was gay, and was openly gay from the beginning of his recovery. He had an edgy, dry sense of humor and was perfectly capable of being irreverent . . . about some of the dogma in AA. I met Barry's life partner, Spencer B., early in my recovery. Spence was one of the first gay people I encountered when I started going to Al-Anon meetings and he was always very encouraging and supportive. Barry and Spence were open, visible, and active [in AA and Al-

Anon] and were an important couple in my life and in the birthing of gay recovery in New York.

Barry and I both wanted to know everybody, and Barry knew vast numbers of people. I decided at my second or third meeting that I was not going to sit in the back of the room and watch other people get sober. *I am going to be a participant in my own recovery,* I thought; it was a rare moment of clarity. *[Laughing]* But here and there, I'd have these little blinding moments of revelation, for all I know, they could have been [my brain] synapses dying! I was just so shocked to feel well that things began to get my attention.

I had a similar experience when I first encountered AA. The environment was such a shock. In 1980 I was living in Sacramento and a friend convinced me to drive to San Francisco with her to attend a planning meeting for the Living Sober conference. At one point, some of the committee members began to disagree. I remember sinking into my folding chair, waiting for the brawl to start. But it never did. No one threw chairs. No one cursed. No one even raised their voice. I had never seen a group of people—much less other gay *people—resolve conflict in such a respectful way.*

Isn't that amazing? I've sat through thousands of AA meetings and planning meetings for AA activities where all kinds of divergent opinions were expressed with a great deal of tolerance and acceptance.

At the first planning meeting for what eventually became the International Advisory Council of Homosexual Men and Women in Alcoholics Anonymous [IAC], there was a contingent of militant lesbian feminist separatists. They arrived angry at this fellow's apartment and within five minutes made it clear that they would not speak directly to any of the men or respond to any of their questions.

Here was this huge barrier of declared hostility, and I got in the middle of it. I supported their right to be angry and to decline to interact with the men in a process designed and governed by men. Well, I say process, but it wasn't as though somebody sat down and wrote out a plan. A bunch of us just got together in this guy's apartment to talk about how to lobby the AA General Service Office to create a committee for gays.

None of those women thanked me for taking their side. They knew I was obviously not one of them, no matter what I tried to say, and the guys felt I was being disloyal. *[Laughing]* A couple of people even suggested [that] I had some serious clinical issues, which may have not been far off the mark either! But, for all of that, there was no yelling, no screaming, no threatening, and eventually we worked it through.

The goal was to organize, so you could approach AA with a proposal for a gay council?

Yes. At the time, gay [AA] groups were emerging all over the place, but we didn't know how to find one another, and we didn't know how to refer people [to gay meetings]. We also saw the need for an acknowledgment of gay and lesbian people in the AA literature. There was a very active Young People's Advisory Council [in AA]. So we thought, *Let's get an International Advisory Council on gays, too.*

I've spoken with several people who were involved in this effort, and each of them recalled one particular meeting where the council's name was being discussed. Were you there?

Oh my god. Yes. Now, you need to put this into context. This was the period when lesbians were organizing, and claiming their rights, not only as gay people, but their rights within the gay movement itself. It was a very painful period in the gay social justice movement because gay men had assumed leadership and didn't cede much of it very easily. They didn't understand that you could be oppressed *and* a sexist, too!

For example, there was a huge battle going on among the organizers of the gay parade in New York because some women had had the nerve to propose that lesbians be allowed to lead the parade on some years, and the men weren't having it! They thought if it weren't for them, there wouldn't be a parade, and all this kind of BS.

In the discussion about creating an advisory committee, what was in sharp focus was whether the word "Men" or the word "Women" should come first in the title, not whether we should call ourselves

"Homosexuals," or "Gays," or whatever. That's where the quarrels were.

Nancy T. mentioned that some people wanted transgendered alco- holics to be reflected in the name as well.

I don't remember that, but she may well be correct. There was at that time a fellow in AA, one of the founders of the New Group, whose name was Padric McG. Padric cross-dressed sometimes. He had long flaming red hair, and wore lots of jewelry and rayon pant- suits. I never thought of him as being transsexual or transgendered, but perhaps he would have. Padric was who he was, and very flam- boyantly so. He was very active in gay AA in New York in the 1970s and 1980s. He might well have been at one of those planning meet- ings.[2]

I grew up in an era when few gay people were visible, and those who were weren't necessarily heroes and role models. It's been terrific to discover how many lesbians and gay men, and now transgendered and bisexual people, have made significant contributions to improv- ing opportunities for gay people with substance abuse problems. Cer- tainly one of the great pioneers is Dr. Max Schneider. He has treated thousands of people, and provided many of the basic education tools used in alcoholism treatment.

Growing up gay when I did, it was almost impossible to feel that anyone valued my life much. It was clear that quite a few people would rather I didn't exist or, if I insisted on existing, that I at least keep my mouth shut about it. I didn't feel welcome in the world. I didn't feel [that] I belonged. AA gave me a place to belong.

In the 1970s, there weren't many places a gay person could go to, to be in a supportive environment, and AA provided that. Gay people in AA helped me recognize that although I had come out, I was bitter and very, very angry. I felt I'd been given the shaft because I'd been made to be gay.

In sobriety, I had the support to gradually go through the coming- out process all over again, and, this time, to choose it. [The people in AA] taught me how to value my life, how to make choices that sup- ported the goals I chose, how to form relationships in a healthy way. I'd never had access to a process that would do that.

It was like having an enormous weight lifted off me, after a lifetime of struggling to drag it around. It was finally okay to be me. In fact, it was perfectly fine to be me! Finally I had a home, a family, and a community.

Chapter 10

New Jersey

Kitty M.

[Kitty was born in Mountain Lakes, New Jersey.]

I was twenty-five in 1957, and living in Columbus, Ohio. I was desperate, drinking heavily, and suicidal. A friend took me to my first AA meeting. The woman closest to me in age [at the meeting] was about fifty. . . . I stayed off alcohol [for about nine months], but I was cross-addicted to prescription medication and didn't know what that did to you. I went back to drinking and drank for another thirteen years.

In 1970, I was teaching at a college about fifty miles south of Washington DC. One February weekend I went to my parents' house in New Jersey and got very drunk, and called a friend in the program.

That summer I came to New Jersey and started going to meetings. Ridgewood, New Jersey, was very upscale, very heterosexual, and very suburban.

Then, in 1974, Sarah came to work where I was working, and I was smitten. *[Laughing]* I was still trying to go straight. I wouldn't have sought out a gay AA meeting if my life [had] depended on it! I didn't want anything to do with all this. So I really was caught. I knew I was gay, but I didn't want to be, and I was miserable.

Sarah and I became fast friends. She was very involved in AA, and I got reinvolved and finally came off all of the pills. We were falling in love, and Sarah was still married, which was difficult. We finally

The History of Gay People in Alcoholics Anonymous
Published by The Haworth Press, Inc., 2007. All rights reserved.
doi:10.1300/5699_10

got together in 1975. At that point she and her husband were getting a divorce.

We went to our first gay meeting in 1976, in Caldwell, New Jersey, and it was thrilling! I was scared. I'd never been to one before, and I didn't know what to expect. [The group] was predominantly gay men. Sometimes issues on the edge of the meeting would come up, like people cruising, and that they shouldn't be doing that, and this was a new phenomenon to me. I grew up in the suburbs, in a totally straight environment, struggling to fit in, and to suddenly find this was wild! It shook me up a lot. It was also the first time since getting sober that I told my real story. People say being in AA is like coming home, but telling my full story at a gay meeting for the first time was my real coming home.

We continued to go to mainstream AA as a primary source. There was some long-term sobriety in the gay meetings, but not a lot. In fact, a lot of it was ours! So it was an iffy business. You go to a gay meeting because you need support, but you are also going for your sobriety. Another thing that disturbed me was the come-and-go quality of the gay meetings. A lot of people came for while and then dropped out.

We were extremely closeted. This was suburban New Jersey. In part, we were protecting Sarah's children, who lived with us. She didn't want her husband coming after us for custody, and there was a real fear that he might take them away.

Today, I go to [both] gay and straight meetings. I want the mix. I want people who have all kinds of life experiences! The breadth of experience in mainstream AA is much greater. The people who taught me the most in straight AA were the men, not because I'm real butch, but because I was a career person. I was a single, independent woman, and I identified with the men who went to work [outside the home]. And so did I.

Trying to get sober in 1958 was extremely difficult because I was a woman, never mind that I was a lesbian! Trying to find a kindred spirit was well nigh impossible. I was in college in the 1950s, and those were miserable times, miserable. Being a lesbian was forbidden. Those years were the very beginning of the movement, when the Mattachine Society and the Daughters of Bilitis first appeared, but there was no place to go with it. I didn't want to be one, and I drank a lot over it—not to be. Later, in 1970, it was very hard. Not many people were out. It was years before my recovery was connected with my lesbian identity.

One last question, Kitty. Have there been people who've been heroes or role models for you in sobriety?

The woman I followed into AA later became my sponsor. I think she had trouble with my being a lesbian sometimes, but she was always there. For a lesbian hero, [sociologist] Lillene Fifield is a hero of mine. Lillene was out, and she was out there doing the work! [Gay Rights Movement leader] Barbara Gittings and [Alcoholism Center for Women cofounder] Brenda Weathers are also my heroes. Another is the woman who took me to my first meeting. She wasn't in need of recovery, but she really helped out.

If you really want to know my hero, it's Sarah. She was the one who confronted me about my drug use. So in some ways, I really owe her my life. So she's my ultimate hero!

Sarah G.

[Sarah grew up in Bergen County, New Jersey.]

In 1971, I was a suburban housewife with three children, living in Franklin Lakes, New Jersey. We'd moved numerous times in the years I was married and had just moved to New Jersey from Illinois. My drinking had really increased and I called a psychiatrist for help. The psychiatrist happened to be seeing a young client whose parents were in AA, and with their permission, he gave me the name of the child's mother. She took me to my first meeting.

Soon after I got sober, I went back to school to get my undergraduate degree. I was very involved in AA, and my husband got involved in Al-Anon. We used to go out speaking together—kind of a Mr. and Mrs. AA and Al-Anon! We were part of a group of about ten couples in recovery. My husband and one other man were in Al-Anon. All the rest of the Al-Anons were women, and I was friends with all the [AA] husbands. The AA women I knew were all suburban housewives, and they weren't exactly role models for me. I wasn't very happy as a housewife. I never really felt like I fit in.

I began working at a little psychotherapy center, and that's where I met Kitty. *[Laughing]* I was going to inform all the therapists there about AA and alcoholism! We got to talking, and we got to be friends, and then we fell in love. This was quite a shock. Although I'd questioned my sexual identity, I had never acted on it before.

I knew that if I was going to stay sober, I was going to have to begin to deal with my life more realistically. I began separating from my husband. Kitty began to work in the alcoholism field. I was getting my master's degree. I was working, plus [I had] three kids at home. It was a pretty crazy time for all of us.

At the time, people in [AA in] Bergen County, New Jersey, didn't think gays should have their own meetings. I had an AA friend who would drive by the gay meetings to see who was going in and who was coming out. So gay meetings weren't the safest place if you didn't want anyone to know you were gay. The straight people knew where [the meetings] were and would stake them out. I was afraid of being discovered and having a child custody problem.

One of the hard things was to have a secret and be going to AA, where everything was about honesty and openness. My whole relationship with AA changed. . . . In 1974, being separated or divorced was not popular. People couldn't understand me changing my sexuality, and that became a threat to many of the people I knew. To begin to deal with my relationship with Kitty was a very positive and happy part of my life, but it was a big secret with AA.

I didn't know any women who worked, or who went to school, or who did anything other than their wifely duties. People used to say to me, "You say you're depressed? If you're depressed, go home and clean your floors and do your windows." What a shock it was to hear a woman at an AA meeting in New York who'd never been married or had children talk about her life. I'd always had this idea that if I hadn't gotten married I would have been able to escape alcoholism. I realized then that if I'd lived her life I probably would have ended up a drunk—just as I had been a drunk housewife in the suburbs. But I had to go into New York to hear an AA speaker like that!

I remember going to the first Big Apple Roundup [the annual gay AA conference] in New York, and thinking, *We live in New Jersey, but we might as well be in Kansas.* At that first Roundup we met people with long-term sobriety from all over. One man had driven up from Florida! They put on a musical that was incredible; there was singing and dancing. It was a very powerful experience.

A real turning point was when my ex-husband said he wanted the children, and they went to live with him, and we moved to New York City. There we were much more open and able to be who we wanted to be. I was working on my PhD and Kitty was working full-time.

Have you had any heroes or role models in recovery, Sarah?

Kitty has been the biggest hero in my life. When I used to get into a fight with my ex-husband, I'd go to an AA meeting. After being with my AA friends a while, I'd forget what I was mad about. We'd talk it through, and I'd go home and I'd be all right. But the first time Kitty and I got into a tangle I was ready to leave and she said, "You can't leave now! You stay here. We're going to talk about this." [Kitty] helped me learn to deal directly with people, not to run away from problems, but to talk about them.

Not to mention the experience of meeting her, and falling in love, of really having an intimate relationship, which I never had with my husband. Working together has been a wonderful part of our lives, and it's been there since the beginning. [Kitty and Sarah have collaborated personally and professionally during their thirty-year partnership.]

We've had this whole experience of sharing, writing, thinking, and formulating things. Being married to your best friend—now, that's having it all!

Chapter 11

We Never Looked Back:
A Conversation with NALGAP
Cofounders Drs. Dana Finnegan
and Emily McNally

Introduction

Drs. Dana Finnegan and Emily McNally are the authors of two groundbreaking books on addiction in the LGBT community, *Dual Identities: Counseling Chemically Dependent Gay Men and Lesbians,* published in 1987, and the recently revised and expanded *Counseling Lesbian, Gay, Bisexual, and Transgender Substance Abusers: Dual Identities.*

In 1979, they cofounded the National Association of Lesbian and Gay Addiction Professionals (NALGAP). NALGAP confronts homophobia and heterosexism in the delivery of addiction services to lesbian, gay, bisexual, and transgendered (LGBT) people and advocates for LGBT-affirming programs. It provides information, training, advocacy, and support for addiction professionals, individuals in recovery, and others concerned about LGBT health.

NALGAP was born at the Rutgers Summer School of Alcohol Studies. Drs. Finnegan and McNally taught their groundbreaking course "Alcoholism and Sexual Identity" at the Summer School from 1981 to 1991. The Summer School attracts students from around the world and many graduates have gone on to do pioneering work in the field of addiction treatment, education, and research.

The History of Gay People in Alcoholics Anonymous
Published by The Haworth Press, Inc., 2007. All rights reserved.
doi:10.1300/5699_11

Dr. Finnegan

In 1979, Emily and I went to the Summer School of Alcohol Studies at Rutgers University. We were petrified someone was going to find out that we were together. In fact, when we weren't both accepted as students on the same day we got paranoid and decided they'd found out we were gay! But we were both accepted, and our experiences there changed our lives, and we never looked back.

We attended the special presentation Nancy T. and Cade W. had been making at the Summer School for a number of years on issues affecting gay and lesbian alcoholics, and that evening Emily noticed a little announcement on the bulletin board of the dorm we were staying in. There was to be a meeting that night of professionals interested in gay and lesbian issues, and it gave a room number in the dorm.

We went to the meeting that night, terrified that we were going to be found out. As I recall, I didn't want to take the elevator *[laughing]* because I was afraid people would know I was going to that meeting when I got out on that floor! I think Emily said, "I have to go to the bathroom. I'll come up in a little while." So we both resisted it in our own way, but we went.

There were fifteen to twenty people there. Here were all these *people!* Most of them were gay or lesbian; a couple of people were bisexual. I'd never met a bisexual person before in my whole life, and I remember not believing them either. I thought they were gay!

That night, Nancy talked to us: "Cade and I are AA members. We can only speak as AA members, as helpful as that may be. People come up to us after the seminar and say, 'I have a client who's gay. What should I do?' We can't tell them what to do! It's not our profession! *You* are the professionals. You are the ones who should be teaching and training other professionals how to work with lesbians and gay men." And she was right.

They talked to us about the need for information. Nancy told us about the directory of services and the list of gay AA meetings she was distributing. You know, she's the ninth wonder of the world. She'd been clipping articles and following journals; she had quite a collection. "You really ought to do something," she said. "It's up to you."

We met a lot during those three weeks, and it was very intense. I hadn't had the privilege of spending time with people who were gay or lesbian. It was like sitting around the campfire, this time with the right people, and being able to tell the truth. We shared our stories with the group. Many of the people in the group were in recovery and telling their real stories for the first time, too.

We talked about what we were going to do. We needed a national organization, and this organization needed an address, and guess who volunteered for that? Emily and I went home to the small town we lived in and got a post office box. It felt very dangerous and daring, although nobody bothered us. We took with us the names of those first fourteen people, who had all of a sudden joined the National Association of Gay Alcoholism Professionals. It was NAGAP then; the "L" wasn't added until later.

We learned [that] the way to start an organization is to *say* you're an organization. We wrote letters to the director of addiction services in every state. We wrote to everyone we could think of. We created a directory of service providers who were, or claimed to be, gay-sensitive. I don't know where she got all this information, but Nancy just opened her files and said, "Here, take this. You are the people who should be doing this." The bibliography, her directory of facilities and services, all of it—we took over the task of collecting and maintaining the information.

A lot of what was in the bibliography was what is referred to as "fugitive" literature.[1] Sometimes there were journal articles, but a lot of [the materials] were papers [that] people had written and presented at a conference, and [then] passed on to others. Brenda Weathers was the first person to address a national conference about what it was like to be gay or lesbian and to be addicted.

Meetings for lesbians and gay men, the so-called "special interest" meetings, are invaluable because they allow people to be completely honest about who they are. That is crucially important for a lot of people [who are] forming and claiming their identity as a lesbian or gay recovering person. That's not true for everybody, though. It's been my experience that some people don't want [to go] or feel the need to go to lesbian or gay meetings. For others, I think having an AA support group that is open and accepting of who you are is essential to recovery—both from addiction and from being stigmatized as gay or lesbian.

How can straight AA members be better allies to gay people and role models for other straight members of their group?

I think that is crucially important. One of the most helpful and positive things we have found is that sometimes a straight person can give more validation than a gay or lesbian person. Emily did her dissertation on lesbian recovering alcoholics in AA and she found that many of them had straight sponsors who were very important to them.

Straight people have a lot of supportive power they don't often know they have. Sometimes a straight person saying you're okay is more powerful than a gay person [saying the same thing] because when a gay person says it you might think, *Well, but what do* you *know. You're just a second-class citizen like me.*

We are all left with our own inner homophobia. I grew up believing that straight people were better than gay people, and even now, many, many, many years later, it still packs a certain punch. A straight person saying, "Go for it!" is a very powerful validation.

The problem was, Where could you send a gay person for treatment that was safe? In the earliest days, we'd call one another.

"I have somebody going into treatment. Do you know anyone, or any place, that's safe?" And someone would say, "Oh! I know, Joe So-and-So is working over here. Let's tell him we're sending someone over." Then Joe—who wasn't out at work himself, remember—could make contact with that person so he'd have a gay liaison—someone watching out for him there, who knew the ropes, who could let him know he wasn't alone.

Early NALGAP member Dr. Michael Picucci

Dr. McNally

Nancy and Cade had been reading the papers they'd written about what it was like to be gay and to be in recovery at the Rutgers Summer School for several years. Nancy later told us that their workshop was usually held the last week of the session. But in 1978 they'd met a woman who'd been running back to her room to call her lover, the whole time she was at the Summer School, because she didn't know any other people there who were gay. So Nancy asked the person in charge of scheduling to put their workshop in the first week, so the gay and lesbian people would have an opportunity to meet each other.

[In 1979], on the third day of the Summer School, she and Cade had held their workshop, and that night [Dana and I] noticed a little note on the dormitory bulletin board: "Gay Professionals Meeting tonight. Room 614."

Dana told you about some of our agonizing [moments] over that meeting, Part of it was because Rutgers University is in New Jersey, so we were away from home, but not very far! But we were desperate to meet other people.

Listening to everyone tell their stories [that night] was a powerful experience. Some of them had never been in a room with another gay person. Some of them had never said out loud that they were gay. That really began the whole NALGAP idea. Nancy had planted the seed, but professionals needed other professionals who were willing to take a risk and come out, to present the materials that would be helpful to other counselors, and to be there for them.

So we kept meeting, and we came up with the name. We each chipped in twenty dollars, and Dana and I went home and formulated the initial activity to get the organization going. People who had done this kind of thing before gave us help. I think it was L____, or George [M.] who told us, "All you have to do to be a national organization is to say you are [a national organization]. You have a constituency!"

We got a post office box and we had some letterhead made up. We met with George at the National Council on Alcoholism [NCA]. We went to a conference where Emery Hetrick spoke. Emery was the first psychiatrist to come out professionally. There, we met Tom Rooney, who was instrumental in the beginning of NALGAP. Tom was voted counselor of the year by the Virginia Alcoholism Association. One of the most wonderful stories I've ever heard was about a woman who read about Tom in the [news]paper and brought her child to see him. She saw that he must be a good counselor if he was voted counselor of the year. She didn't care whether he was gay or not! Emery died from AIDS. A lot of the pioneers have—Cade W., Tom Ziebold, and Tom Mongen.

I had thousands of three-by-five cards containing the names and addresses of the places we were sending information—treatment centers, state directors, NCA. There was a woman in Oklahoma named Patricia Zigrang, who was running a group for gay men at a veterans' hospital. At one point, Patricia left Oklahoma, and I remember having to take the entire state off the facilities and services list because one person was all there was. When Patricia moved, the whole state disappeared!

In 1981, Dana and I began a course at the Summer School called "Alcoholism and Sexual Identity." We team-taught it with Tom Rooney and a number of other teachers because it was important to have both gay men and lesbians recognized. [Many of the students] at the school were there on scholarships from the military. The Catholic church sent a lot of priests and nuns, and we had people from other countries. Many of them had nowhere else to go to talk about some of the things that had happened to them.

One person had once been accused of being gay and it had traumatized him. He didn't know what to do with that experience. One year we had a gay priest who was attending the Summer School with his partner, and in the same group, we had a lesbian who had gone to confession as an adolescent and been told by the priest that she was a sinner, and had lived most of her life in agony. Many of the students became very close, since they were all thrown into the middle of all this.

[Every year], on the last day of the Summer School, there was a big dance. The first time [Dana and I] went, the gay people all stood around on the outside and watched. Then they went back to their rooms, or out to a gay bar [to dance]. The next year, Dana and I started to dance. Soon, other people joined us, and soon the dance became a wonderful part of the Summer School.

It was quite an inspiration, and we have met some wonderful people [at the Summer School]. Once in a while, someone will come up to us and say, "I was at the Rutgers Summer School. It changed my life."

Chapter 12

San Francisco

Introduction

Over in Oakland I knew of a bar where you could dance. You had to climb up a fire escape, and go past a security guard, who had to know somebody in your group, before you could get in. . . .

Down in Sharp Park there was a bar called Hazel's; there weren't many places like this, but these were places that paid off the cops, so it was okay. One Sunday, I missed going to Hazel's, just by a fluke, and that afternoon they backed up six army trucks, and anybody who was dancing was hauled off to jail.

The next morning the front page of the *Chronicle* listed their names, addresses, and place of employment—the whole thing. Many of those people lost their jobs.

Don K.

In February 1956, Sheriff Whitmore of San Mateo County and his staff, assisted by military police, the California Highway Patrol, and agents from the state Alcoholic Beverage Control Board, rounded up nearly 300 people at Hazel's Bar. Ninety of them were arrested and charged with vagrancy.

In 1959, the California Supreme Court affirmed the right of homosexual women and men to congregate in public when it ruled that the Alcoholic Beverage Control Board could not revoke a business's liquor license simply because homosexuals were known to gather there (Boyd 2003).

The History of Gay People in Alcoholics Anonymous
Published by The Haworth Press, Inc., 2007. All rights reserved.
doi:10.1300/5699_12

Gordon T.

I moved to San Francisco in 1959. It was a great place for night-clubs and drinking. I fit right in! . . . I had a group of friends, and we went to the bars and to parties. We went to the opera. We drank before the opera, and we drank after the opera. There was a man in the group I ran with, named Burke, who'd gone to Alcoholics Anonymous [AA]. *[Laughing]* We all knew about it because we gossiped about him! I saw him drinking at a party one time and I thought, *Oh, that's wonderful. Look. AA has taught him how to control his drinking.*

I started working at an oil company, in the data-processing department. They didn't object to my drinking; my boss and the people around me drank too, but when I started working the graveyard shift it really got out of control. [One] weekend [in particular] started out like most others.

I got off work at eight [o'clock] on Saturday morning and went and had drinks; I probably went to a brunch. That night I remember playing cards with some friends and drinking till I fell off my chair. They put me to bed, and it was all all right; they didn't object because they drank too. Sunday, it was another round of bars, and at around eight [o'clock that night] I realized I wasn't going to make it to work at midnight, so I thought, *I'll call Burke, and see about this AA.* Well, calling someone at eight o'clock to find out how to save the job you're going to lose at midnight is kind of stupid, but I did it anyway.

I found out that Burke was back in AA. He said he'd take me to a meeting the next day if I would go the entire day without drinking. It was very difficult, but I did it, and I went to work that night. [Monday] evening a friend of his picked me up to take me to [an AA] meeting in Sausalito, and on the way we stopped at Zak's [Restaurant], where we met other people having dinner before the meeting. At the Gratitude Group, in Sausalito, I was introduced to the secretary, who told me, "Gordon, with the help of AA, you don't ever have to drink as long as you live, if you don't want to." Of course, I thought that was kind of strange, not to want to drink.

It was a mixed group, gay and straight. They were all nicely dressed, elegant people from good walks of life. One was the owner of a gay bar. One woman was an interior decorator, and there was a very elegantly dressed, handsome man who had been an assistant to

Governor Jerry Brown. It was nice, you know, and I decided I would give this AA thing a try.

My thinking went something like this: *If I am going to lose my job, I'll lose all my junk that is in hock. A lot of my friends are kind of avoiding me at the parties I want to go to, and in six months it will be Christmas. If I don't lose my job, with all the money I don't spend on gin, I can get my stuff out of hock, and then, when people see how nice I am, not falling down drunk anymore, I will be invited to all the Christmas parties, and I will be able to start drinking again.*

Burke recommended that we go to a meeting every day for the first week, and at least two meetings a week after that, and I figured that I could go to the movies on the off nights. Burke had dragged me around and introduced me to a lot of people, including all the gay people he knew in AA. And the night I'd planned to go to the movies, I found out there was another meeting some of my new friends were going to, and I wanted to be there, too.

At the Monday Beginners Group, they were electing a new coffee maker, and the outgoing coffee maker asked if I would take over for him. Roland and I are still good friends. We always joke that he can't get drunk because then I'll have more sobriety than he will! The two of us that held the coffee maker position at the Monday Beginners Group in 1967 are still sober today.

I found out that a lot of the gay people from that meeting did service at the meeting at St. Mark's, and that most of them went over to Miz Brown's [Coffee Shop] and had ice cream and chatted there afterward. I always wanted to be invited, and once in a while they did invite me. But after a couple of times, I found out that I didn't need to be invited. I could just go! And then I found out that I could invite people to Miz Brown's.

I met a lot of people I really liked in AA. I was still going to bars with my old friends once in a while, and they were awfully nice to me. I remember having brunch with them one day and realizing that I was really not part of [the group], that I really didn't belong, and that the only way to be a part of [that group] was to drink. But I didn't want to stay until Christmas [when I planned to start drinking again], so I got up and left.

Soon it was Christmas, and I found I'd been right. I got all my junk out of hock, and then I got a lot more junk. . . . My job was going well, and I got invitations to a lot of Christmas parties. Things were going so well, I decided to try and stay sober, and so far, I've been able to. I always say, "I never quit drinking; I'm just not drinking today," and that has worked very well.

In those days AA had a big [Christmas] dinner dance at the Palace Hotel. That was kind of grand, you know. . . . The Under Thirty-Five Group over in North Beach was mostly all gay people, and we all bought tickets. . . . There was a woman who always came to that meeting, and she had a ticket too, so our table had nine men and one woman!

People in [AA] in San Francisco were always very accepting of the gay people. They didn't say, "Oh, *you* can't be here," or anything [like that]. Gay people did a lot of AA service work, things people with kids don't always have the extra time to do. One time a woman complained to Central Office that all the people in service at Monday Beginners were gay, and they just ignored it.

I felt comfortable being a gay person in AA. I didn't feel out of place, though a couple of people did. There was one fellow in particular who was having a hard time staying sober. He used to say, "If we had a meeting where gay people could talk any way that we wanted to, I know I could stay sober."

In 1967, . . . I gave a little party and invited everyone I knew in AA that was gay. We held a vote by secret ballot on whether to have a gay meeting, and we asked people to indicate whether they would support it or not. Some people said they didn't think we needed a gay meeting. Others said we needed one, but that they would not support it. But the majority opinion was that we needed one anyway, and we decided that the next week we would have one.

My downstairs neighbors offered their apartment for the first meeting, but there was a fellow there that night from New York, who said they'd tried to start a couple of gay meetings in New York in private apartments, but that they hadn't worked out because personalities got involved. So we decided the best thing would be to meet in a church, or other public place with no personal affiliations.

We tried to think of a place and came up with many suggestions. One friend, a member of the Episcopal church on Fell Street, said he thought that would be a good place because the priest had said all people were welcome there. He made an appointment for me with the pastor and he said, "Yes." The following week, in February 1968, we met at the church.

People had put the word out all around, and, my god! People came out of the woodwork! People I never knew were even interested in AA! We elected a secretary, and I was elected treasurer. At that time, the San Francisco Central Office would not list us in the meeting directory or accept our Seventh Tradition donations. . . . So I sent the money to the General Service Office in New York.

Since we weren't listed by the Central Office, we put a classified ad in the *Berkeley Barb* that said, "Gay? Drinking problem? Need help? Call . . ." and I had my phone number listed, so that when people called I could tell them about the meetings. There were maybe ten to twenty people for the first year or two at the Fell Street Group. There were some people who didn't want to be identified as being gay, so they didn't come in the beginning, or, if they came, they wouldn't participate much. But with time people became more trusting.

There were almost no women in AA that we knew of who were out at that time, a few maybe, but they didn't seem to be interested [in coming to the meeting]. There was one girl who showed up one day—she was very butch—and we didn't know if it was a girl or a boy. We didn't want to exclude anybody who was willing to take part, but there were some in the group who didn't want any women, or any street people, or anything else. So the meetings were for gay men alcoholics only.

Some of us didn't like the idea that women weren't welcome. We didn't want to lose anyone that came around, and in late 1968, we started a group for men and women down at the Gay Community Center.[1] That meeting soon moved because a lot of people didn't want to go south of Market Street. At that time, it was very dangerous. Not long after that, the Fell Street Group opened up to all people. The Post and Mason Group was another early gay meeting [that] met for a while at Glide Memorial Baptist Church.

Now we live in Hawaii. . . . In Waikiki, we have a meeting at seven o'clock in the morning called Twelve Coconuts. There's a circle of twelve coconut palms on the beach, and people sit beneath the trees and have a meeting. We get anywhere from twenty to a hundred people, and I'm pretty regular there. . . .

A few months ago, I had a heart attack. My doctor sent me to the emergency room, and then I had heart bypass surgery. I was in the intensive care unit for three days.

When I came to, there was a nurse standing over me. "Hey," he said, looking down at me. "You're Gordon. From Coconuts!"

He was my nurse every night for the next three nights. It's very nice to know that you have someone taking care of you who is clean and sober.

A Safe and Central Place to Meet

In the 1960s, it was almost impossible to find a church that would permit a group of homosexuals to meet on the premises. The ease with which the founders of the AA Fell Street Group found a safe and central place to meet is due to the efforts of an organization called "CRH," San Francisco's Council on Religion and the Homosexual.

In 1964, a man named Ted McIlvenna was the director of the Young Adult Project at Glide United Methodist Church in the Tenderloin. McIlvenna was disturbed by the numbers of homeless gay youth he saw on the streets, kids who'd been tossed out of their homes when their parents discovered that they were gay. McIlvenna and Lewis Durham, of Glide's Urban Foundation, arranged a meeting between local religious leaders and representatives from San Francisco's homophile community to talk about these and other issues facing gay people at that time. In 1964, sixteen ministers from local Methodist, Episcopal, Lutheran, and Quaker churches met with leaders from the Daughters of Bilitis, the Mattachine Society, the League for Civil Education, and San Francisco's Tavern Guild, a group of gay tavern owners. And in December of that year the Council on Religion and the Homosexual (CRH) was founded.

The CRH was very active in the fight for gay people's rights. Its members were the first to proclaim that all people were welcome to join their congregations (a euphemism used by churches to this day that means "everybody, plus homosexuals"). The CRH sponsored symposiums on homosexuality and supported the candidates' nights organized by San Francisco's homophile groups. They published and distributed a pamphlet called *Every Tenth Person Is a Homosexual* (McAdams n.d.; D'Emilio 1998).

Each of the San Francisco churches that opened their doors to gay AA groups in the late 1960s and early 1970s had clergy who were active in the CRH. These included the Episcopal Church of the Advent (261 Fell Street); Glide United Methodist; the United Church of Christ's First Congregational Church (432 Mason Street at Post); and Trinity Episcopal Church (1668 Bush at Gough). Many of those early gay AA groups continue to meet in their original locations today.

In 1969, the first gay AA group in Southern California held their first meeting in Los Angeles at the Metropolitan Community Church (MCC). At the time services were held in the home of Reverend Troy Perry, MCC's founder. MCC churches around the world continue to provide safe, supportive, accessible meeting space for gay, lesbian, bisexual, and transgendered members of twelve-step programs.

Tony P.

[Tony got sober in San Francisco in January 1964.] I understand you were a regular at many of the San Francisco AA groups frequented by gays and lesbians in the 1960s—groups like the Under Thirty Five Group in North Beach, the Telegraph Hill Group, and the Gratitude Group in Sausalito. Were you aware that there were homosexuals at those meetings?

At some point I became aware of it. I've never had a gay experience, so I didn't have any conscious feeling about identifying gays, or thinking that someone was gay. Let me tell you a little story.

When my first AA sponsor moved to Oakland, he told me I ought to find a new sponsor. So I looked around, and one day I met this fellow named Norman W. from the Telegraph Hill Group. Norm said he'd be glad to be my sponsor and he suggested we have dinner and go to a meeting every week together, and I thought that was a great idea.

Norm was one of the greatest people I'd ever met. He was just so charming, and good-looking. He'd been sober about five years then, and was a really spiritual person. Norman was just the perfect second sponsor for me. At that time I was about to get married. I'd asked my girlfriend, my wife now, if she would marry me, and she'd said yes. She had a roommate, named Gloria, who was really a wonderful woman.

One night, after about a month of having dinner and going to a meeting together, Norm and I came out of the old Alano Club on Grant Avenue and started walking to the garage.

"Norm," I said, "there's been something I wanted to talk to you about. My wife-to-be has this roommate named Gloria, and she is absolutely wonderful. She'd be a perfect match for you."

[Norm said,] "What?"

"Yes!" I went on, "Boy, if you could be with her, and date her, we could be a foursome. It would really be great. Because she's intelligent, she's charming, and she's spiritual."

It was pouring down rain that night and Norman gently pushed me under an awning. "Tony," he said, "surely you don't—Don't you know I'm gay?"

"No," I said, "I didn't know that. But look, Norman. I want to tell you something. If you'd just go out with Gloria, if you'll just start dating her, you'll forget all about this gay stuff, whatever it is."

Norm looked at me kind of baffled. I don't think he'd ever met anybody as stupid as I was.

He said, "Tony, I don't want to change. I'm a gay man, and I want to stay gay."

"Oh," I said. "I'm very sorry. I didn't know that's the way it worked."

"Well, that's the way it's worked with me, Tony. So let's not have any more of this. Let's talk about this more later, and I'll tell you more about the gay lifestyle, and the things we do."

So Norm really taught me about gay people—because I had no clue, not a clue.

One of the best illustrations of this was when, about mid-1965, he said, "I'm going to start a gay AA group just for gay people." Well, I hit the roof because, by now, I'm a dedicated AA.

"Norm, we don't belong apart," I said. "We all belong together. If you went to gay groups, I would never have met you. And you never would have become my sponsor."

You know, in the 1960s and 1970s, it was not healthy to be a gay person around. The police raided the bars. Gay people got beat up on the street, even in the Castro, which was even then starting to be gay; people used to come in, just to beat 'em up. A gay bar was a real place for trouble.

Norm said, "Tony, there are a whole bunch of young gay alcoholics out there who don't dare come to straight meetings. I want to start a meeting so they can come in and find out about AA." He was doing this with a couple of his friends. "We're going to tell them that the meeting is to get them acquainted with AA, so they can join the larger AA community."

He had a few good arguments too. "There are women's groups," he said, "and nobody objects to women's groups, so why not have our groups?" That sounded very reasonable to me.

After that, I began to notice some things. At Telegraph Hill, and at the Sausalito meeting, I began to notice that there were gay people there, but it didn't become conscious to me, until Norman educated me. Then I looked for them.

They would say in their sharing sometimes that they were gay, so I learned that way, and then I began to notice that there were gay couples coming in, and that was pretty obvious, even to somebody as stupid as I was. I could tell by the way they'd hold hands and things like that, you know. So I began to get it.

We had a great little Steps study meeting going in Noe Valley, just the other side of the Castro, and one day I noticed that the meeting had started to grow dramatically. There were a lot of people in there! What was happening was that several gay guys had discovered the meeting and were coming regularly. That meeting is now predominantly gay, but it's not advertised as a gay meeting.

I never had the slightest feeling of prejudice of any kind in this matter. I don't know why. I guess [it was] because I was deep into AA when all this occurred. Within the confines of AA, I never experienced the slightest bit of prejudice, but outside AA, in San Francisco, it was not uncommon. I think that it was the spiritual ethics of Alcoholics Anonymous asserting themselves, or itself. I remember several times somebody saying something about some person, like using a term like "faggot," and it was a sure clue to the total isolation of that individual. No one would have anything to do with him after that.

Have you ever sponsored a gay person?

I'm kind of proud of this. I've always had a number of sponsees. And all the time I've been in AA I've always had at least one gay sponsee. I have only one reservation, and I started this with the very first one, who[m] I still sponsor today. I told him that because I was so ignorant of this kind of relationship, I thought he really ought to have dual sponsors, that if he wanted to really confide about his sex life with his partner, he ought to get a gay sponsor to talk to. I felt very uncomfortable not having had that experience personally, and that led me into a broader horizon in my own sobriety.

For example, if I get some felon that I'm sponsoring who's been released from San Quentin—it doesn't happen often, but sometimes I get one, especially since I was a lawyer—I tell them, "If you want to talk about your experiences in prison and your attitudes in prison, you can, but I might have to stop you and say you'd probably be better off talking to an ex-con about that." And that works out very well.

I would like to offer readers some ideas about how they can be more supportive of AA's gay members at meetings. Do you have any thoughts about that?

Whenever anyone with more than a year's sobriety asks me to sponsor them, my first question is, "How many people do you sponsor?" And if I get the answer, "None," I tell them, "What you've got to do is get two sponsees. There are a lot of [new people] coming in [to AA] in San Francisco. Start telling them you'll be their temporary sponsor. Get their phone numbers. Then report back to me, with two sponsees and their phone numbers, and I will be your sponsor." . . .

In fact, I did this just last week. One of these guys is a straight guy, and he said he didn't have any sponsees. I go down to the High Noon Group almost every day—there are lots of gay men and women there—and this fellow and I went to the meeting together.

"Have you got your sponsees yet?" [I asked him.]

"No, I'm working on it," he said.

Well, a young man at the meeting held up his hand and said he had two days [sober].

So I told him, "There's your opportunity!"

"Oh," he said. Then he looked at me. "Tony, I think he's gay."

"Oh, all the better. Man, what an opportunity for you!"

I love doing that! So that gets them off to a good start. If they have any prejudice, it gets them over it pretty fast.

Do you have any final thoughts you'd like to add?

You know, I really don't. There's no separation in my mind anymore about it. That's the reason I was a little reluctant to be interviewed on this whole thing because I don't really see any problem. Is that counterproductive?

Homophobia isn't the issue it used to be in AA, particularly in places like San Francisco or New York. But not so very far outside these cities, attitudes in the larger AA community can be very different.

Prejudice has no place at all in the fellowship of Alcoholics Anonymous. "The only requirement for membership is a desire to stop drinking." That's enough for any of us to have to deal with. This program of Alcoholics Anonymous is God's private property. God is always there, and we declare it when we say *[paraphrasing the Second Tradition]*, "There is only one power, and that is our group conscience, and by following God, as we understand God, in that group conscience." God has no favorites. There is no one so low, or so high, that [he or she] can't be one of God's kids in this fellowship.

Gin B.

[Gin lives in Pacifica, a small town on the coast about thirty minutes south of San Francisco.]

We had a mixed group of friends, about fifteen altogether, half gals and half guys. This was down in Redwood City. We'd navigate up to San Francisco and hit some of the bars—mixed bars [both gay men and women] and bars that were both straight and gay. This was in the post–beatnik era around 1950, up through 1965. We'd go places together, camping, that sort of thing, but it was mostly a home partying scene. It was a heavy drinking crew.

There was a guy in our group who'd joined up with AA, and people honored him when he was on the program. So I knew about AA, but, no, I went pretty much at gunpoint.

In 1964, . . . I had a three-week blackout. Coming home from a party one night I decided to pull over and go to sleep, and I parked on the road down to my place. But I parked in the middle of the road, in the middle of the yellow line, with the motor running. I was in a sports car that didn't have a top. My dog was with me, and when the sheriff came to investigate, she wouldn't let him touch me. So they called the dog pound, to get the pound guy out, so they could get the dog, so they could get me. I didn't know about any of this until the next day, when I got bailed out of Redwood City jail and taken down to Ruth and Pat's place. . . .

Ruth was a partner of mine for twelve years. On Sunday afternoons we usually went out and drank martinis, and that Sunday afternoon they went out and left me with a pile of what turned out to be AA literature. Later I found out why they had all that literature. Pat had been in AA and was on a sabbatical from the program, so they hadn't been collecting it for me.

They left me there by myself. I didn't have a car. The car was impounded. My dog was impounded. Later, they took me to the pound to see if I could get her out. That's when they said, "Would you like to go to an AA meeting tonight?" I felt so bad about her being at the pound that I agreed to go.

Ruthie and I were trying to figure out what to do next. Pat knew the ropes and said she was going to call AA to see if she could find someone for a Twelfth Step call. They got hold of a woman, who turned out to be my first sponsor, a little short Greek gal called Big Connie. Big Connie and a cowboy-type guy came down and dragged me to a meeting. . . .

Back then, they believed in the posse system. They grabbed you by the ear, and you didn't have a chance. If they could keep you standing up and sitting on your chair, you went. If your sponsor didn't take you, one of her posse came and got you.

I'd get a few days [of sobriety] together, sometimes a week or two. Then my sponsor would make me a cake because I was so good, and I'd go out again. I flopped and slid and sloshed around for about eight months, and finally it grabbed hold, in September of 1965. My sponsor told me not to drink between meetings; not to smoke any funny cigarettes, which I didn't like anyway; not to take any funny pills, which I didn't know what they were; and not to get involved emotionally for the first year. So, with three weeks [of sobriety], I ran into another loser.

After meetings she and I would go down to the bowling alley to talk about the meeting, read the book, and have a few drinks. After this woman I'd teamed up with got us kicked out of an apartment in

Redwood City, Ruth and Pat took her in. Then I moved up to Brisbane, and the four of us were under the same roof. She got about four years [of sobriety] together, and was in and out [of AA] after that.

The early 1970s was about the time a gay meeting or two started up in the city. The men started up first, as I recall. The meeting I knew of was at Acceptance House [San Francisco's first halfway house for gay alcoholics]. Most of us knew each other from other meetings in town . . . and, gradually, we had up to fifteen people. But I didn't stick around. It seemed like it was more concentrating on everybody looking everybody else over, and a social sort of thing. So I got back to regular meetings. I went to a lot of meetings south of Market, and I got a home group down there. Once in a while I'd drop in to the meeting on Fell Street; it was primarily guys. In fact, sometimes I felt kind of silly, if there weren't one or two more gals there. . . .

Do you feel more comfortable sharing at a gay meeting than at a regular one?

Not particularly. I talk a lot at the noon meetings here in Pacifica; I just don't get down to all the specifics. People know you're there. They know who you are, and what you are, but you don't bother identifying or talking about it. There are two or three who come occasionally, who'll talk about being lesbian or gay, and it's perfectly acceptable.

We've got all sorts of assorted nuts here in Pacifica, believe me. It's a wonderful mixture of redneck and professional, people who live in the bushes, and you name it. It's a very accepting bunch. If this one says, "My relationship," you know it's his wife. With that one, you know it's the gal he's shacked up with. And if I talk about a relationship, they know what it is. So you can all talk pretty freely.

In the late 1970s, the Uptown Group, my home group, met in the little red church near Market Street. By that time, the Castro had started up, with a boom-boom-bang, and the women's movement was going strong. At Church and Market [Streets], [the Uptown Group] was right at the edge of the Castro, and we would get people in there who wanted to change the book and put "Goddess" in. People didn't want all this stuff going on. We didn't want goddesses floating around in the Big Book![2] So we split. One of the oldest groups in San

Francisco split. The Rebels, as we called them, took over, and the rest of us went up to Twenty-Third Street and became the Home Group. The Rebels weren't necessarily lesbians. I think a lot of them were from the Women's Movement. It was a duke's mixture of anybody that wanted to rebel against anything that moved in there.

In fact, somebody at that meeting scared the livin' bejesus out of me! She came in with a long, black Zorro cape on. She's sort of a grim-looking person anyway, tall, and an artist. She scared me. Judith's not at all that way anymore. She and I have become real good friends. Judith does a lot of work with the homeless. She goes to the really, really south of Market groups, where they fall out of the chairs. She comes down to Pacifica meetings on Fridays. . . .

I moved here because I like Pacifica AA. . . . People discuss anything and everything, but they stick to the program. You can always count on some people being up here *[she raises her hands, thumbs-up, over her head]* and some being down here *[she drops them, thumbs-down]*. Some of them are going to be in the depressed group, and, later, they're with the happy, joyous, and freebies, but they're not all at the same place at the same time. I also like that the age groups are varied. You get some real youngies, to the old dinosaurs, as they call us.

We've got a few around here who are older than I am, but newer in the program, and some of them, if the word "drugs," of any kind, is mentioned, oh boy. Every once in awhile, one of these old codgers will say, "We can't have these druggies at our meetings!" And we have to get them back in line, or they flare up. I was the secretary for a while, and we had one of these guys in there. This guy called out [someone] who mentioned drugs: "This is an AA meeting!" he yelled. "Go to the NA meeting!"

I've got a temper that's, well—I've got a pretty low flashpoint. So after the meeting I was primed for bear. "By God, H____, if these meetings were limited to pure alcoholics, we'd have to meet in a damn phone booth!" I told him. "There ain't no such animal anymore!"

You can figure that, every two or three years, we're going to kick the dead horse around again, but other than that, we're a pretty peaceful group. We get quite a few tourists here too, and city people drop down. Like I say, it's a nice group of assorted nuts. It's the mix that I like.

I have the same trouble with plain old women's meetings. I tried for years to hook into one because I thought, *Gee, I ought to be going to one of those. It would be good for me.* Oh! *[Rolling her eyes, and raising her hand to her forehead like Camille]* Talk about your Al-Anon salute! The drama! Oh, we get the problems, problems out the kazoo. A good AA meeting is about the solution, not the problem. . . .

Is there an experience that stands out in your mind as a defining AA moment for you?

[She reflects for a minute.] One would be my first meeting after my last slip. I was still trying to get rid of the Loser. She'd been out on a run up in the city, and I'd had the sheriff come and evict her. To celebrate that I'd finally got rid of her, I went and got me a jug and just got swacked. The next day she decides she's going to save my soul and yanks me up to a meeting in the city. Then down to [the Alano Club] on Golden Gate, where they're showing the movie *Bill's Story.* . . . She got me to more meetings the next day. She quit drinking long enough to Twelve-Step me. *[She falls silent.]*

Then there were these three gay guys, up in the city, Howard, Bill, and Charlie.

I'd had a big fight with the Loser, and Howard, Bill, and Charlie decided they were going to see to it that I didn't go out. They took turns getting me to meetings. They got me working on the Steps. My first sponsor didn't work with me on the Steps. If I could walk, she dragged me to a meeting, but as far as any coursework, no. I'd been around for eight years sitting on the First Step. I'd gone to a lot of meetings, trying to keep what's-her-face from going out—and if you left her alone for a second, she'd be out—so I had a lot of meetings under my belt, but that was all I had. And when that relationship blew up, I didn't have much to go on.

Howard took it under his skull that he was going to work on that end of things, and he knew he was going to have to do it very subtly. Every Saturday morning we'd meet with our bicycles at the Third Street Bridge in the city, and we'd ride, . . . and all the time, he was working on me.

"Why don't you read this?" he'd say. He had me reading all sorts of Buddhist stuff, and Emmett Fox, a mixture. That went on for about a year, and that's when he said, "The other eleven Steps. Those are the painkillers." And he got me at it. Howard, Bill, and Charlie—they were the turning point.

Charlie died drunk. He never made it. Bill retired and moved to Hawaii. Howard wanted to find the place at the end of the road, away from everything, and everybody, and he looked all over the state of California, and moved to most of them. He finally ended up by the Oregon border in a place called Fort Jones.

Howard was going deaf, and he was one of those guys, who— Dang if he was going to wear a hearing aid! You couldn't carry on a conversation! He'd bounce down here every once in awhile, and we'd be sitting in an AA meeting, where people were talking about some- body's funeral, and Howard would sit there, nodding and smiling, and say, "Oh, that's nice."

One of his sponsees up at Fort Jones moved down to the Santa Cruz mountains. When Howard got a little more racked up, he and his wife brought him down . . . to live with them. They tried all sorts of hearing aids on him, but he won't wear them. We dropped in on them a couple years back, and we just couldn't communicate at all.

They saved my neck—those guys did.

Ruth F.

[Ruth got sober in 1965.]

In 1965, I was living with Pat. She and I were drinkers together, and lovers. Unbeknownst to me, Pat had been in AA ten years earlier. Ridiculously enough, she'd even accused *me* of being an alcoholic.

One Sunday my friend Ginny arrived at our place at seven a.m. af- ter spending the night in jail; she'd been picked up for being drunk. When she got to our house Pat . . . pulled some AA stuff out of a has- sock I didn't even know was there. That evening Ginny went to her first AA meeting. And subsequent to that, a marvelous thing hap- pened. She was only drunk half the time!

When I was sixteen an English teacher got through to me about how marvelous the great writers were, and how they were all nuts. Being sixteen, I checked myself out, and finding myself pretty nutty,

I thought, *This qualifies me to be a great writer.* This necessity to become a great writer flared up from time to time, and that October, during one of these flare-ups, I checked my schedule. I got up in the
morning, went to work, came home, had a couple of drinks, ate dinner, and went to bed. You know, I was *really* busy. I didn't have time
to start my great writing.

I told Pat I was going to quit drinking so I'd have time to write.
"Fine," she said, and, just to put the pressure on, "If you drink, there's
no sex." She really knew how to hurt a person! But it didn't matter
because I wasn't going to drink. It just didn't matter at all, although it
mattered a few days later.

I'd been sober three days and I was doing fine. So if there was any
problem about alcoholism, it wasn't with me. Thursday I stopped at
the liquor store. And as I'm reaching for the bottle of gin this voice in
my head says, "What are you doing buying gin? I thought you weren't
going to drink anymore." But I didn't want to talk to any little voices.
Then the voice changed. "Only an alcoholic has to drink," it said. And
it kept repeating this. "Only an alcoholic has to drink."

I had not had anything to drink for three days, and I had to drink.

When I got home, I opened the bottle and made myself a martini,
loathing myself because I didn't understand about alcoholism. . . . I
was drinking with this terrible knowledge about myself, trying to
fight my way out. A few nights later we went out and ended up at the
No Name Bar in Sausalito, and that turned out to be the last drink either one of us ever had.

[The next day] I talked to Pat. "I've been in bad company, obviously, people who drink too much," I said. "I need to make some new
friends—people who play bridge and chess, and things like that, who
have fun without drinking."

Pat says, "Oh, I know where there are some of those folks."

Well, I am all for this! I want to meet them! So Pat takes me to the
San Francisco Alano Club. It is a perfectly horrid place, as I saw it at
the time. When we got there, nobody was playing bridge or chess.
But they said that a meeting was starting in a few minutes, and did we
want to go? Pat seemed to think it was a good idea, so we went, and it
was really bad. The speaker had had every illness anybody ever heard
of, starting with whooping cough at six weeks old, and finally she had

a hysterectomy, and we were only up to 1940 or so. I never did hear whether she had any problems with alcohol.

The meeting was held up under the roof in the building, with six or seven people around a rectangular table with a big hole in the middle. In those days I was very aware of how much money somebody might or might not have, and these people didn't have any. Third and Mission hadn't gotten cleaned up like it is now; the people who were homeless or really down-and-out lived there. That's where these men had been. After the speaker talked, they talked. They said they were sick, and there was no question in my mind about that. *My god,* I thought. *If I were as sick as they are, I'd get drunk.*

As we left, Pat asked me, with great enthusiasm, how I liked the meeting. Walking out, I had a vision of my future and it was totally empty.

I was in a state of distress greater than anything I've ever felt. I was really dead, but I hadn't gotten horizontal. I am at a point where I have decided that this won't work and that I will have to destroy myself.

My reply was that I didn't think it would work, and I'd just do it myself, but I knew I couldn't do it myself. But I was already trying to distance myself from people who cared about me, see, and there she was.

Now, Pat had two years previously in AA, so she knew what she was hearing. There was a telephone booth right there on the corner, and she . . . called a woman named Ruth S. in Marin County. Ruth remembered Pat. Ruth had been sober a long time, and she wanted to talk to me. Ruth seemed to think it was very important that I go see some woman named Barbara that night in San Francisco, and because it was so important to her, I said I would do it. It's ten o'clock Sunday night, and I'm supposed to go to work in the morning, but none of this mattered anymore.

Pat and I go over and talk to Barbara. I'm pretty sure I almost convinced her I wasn't an alcoholic, but it turned out that Barbara hadn't been to a meeting for a while, and she really needed a meeting, and would really appreciate it if I would just go with her. And since I didn't have anything better to do with my life, what little was left, I agreed to meet Barbara there the next night.

There were a lot of people there. . . . The speaker was a man named Paul G., and that night he described one of the times he'd tried to commit suicide. And I understand an awful lot about this because this is where I am going.

Paul said that, this time, he had decided to gas himself. He blew out the pilot light on the stove, turned on the oven, and stuck his head in, ready to die. Now, Paul was a smoker, and while he was waiting to die, he thought he needed a cigarette. But he postponed it because he was waiting to die. If you've ever been a smoker, you know that when that need [for a cigarette] comes on, it just keeps growing. And it got worse and worse, this need for a cigarette, and, finally, he had to have one. So he went out to the backyard, and had a cigarette because, as he said, "Only a fool would have lit a match in that kitchen."

And I laughed. I understood *exactly* how this was! And I laughed. And within that laughter was a little spark of hope. That's all it was— just a little spark of hope.

After the meeting, Paul told me to try to get to a meeting the next night without taking a drink, and I decided that I would try. I got to a meeting the next night. I was searching frantically for a way not to be an alcoholic, but I couldn't get away from the fact that I'd had three days without a drink. And, as far as I was concerned, with three days of sobriety, I was stone cold sober. That kept me coming back and listening.

Pat wasn't drinking, and I was going to AA without her. She didn't want to drink in front of me, and after a few weeks of this she felt so much pressure that she went to a meeting. When we walked in, a man named Ralph said, "Hi, Ruth. How's your drunken girlfriend?"

"Ralph," I said, "I'd like you to meet Pat." . . . We all laughed, and it cracked the resistance Pat had about going back to AA. Ruth S. had also gotten through to her somewhere in the middle of all of this, so then Pat was there. . . .

Six months later, Ginny ended up getting sober. Gin had a girl-friend named Margo, who was sober sometimes, and not sober sometimes. Margo was cooking for a Catholic nuns' place, in Redwood City. We found out that Margo was on some kind of running drunk, and that a nun was going to go to Ginny's house with the police to get Margo, and put her in some sort of drying-out place. Pat thought we should rescue Margo, before the nun and the police got to her. So we went down and stole Margo and we took her home with us. So when the nun and the police arrived, Margo wasn't there.

After we brought Margo to our house, she quit drinking and the three of us lived in the little house in Brisbane for a while. We also got acquainted with the nun. I felt an obligation to tell her that Margo was safe. So I made an appointment to talk to her.

Sister Anna Marie was very frustrated with us stealing Margo, but she kept her tongue. We had an in-depth conversation about alcoholism. I was new in recovery, and I had a lot of answers.

She told me she was going to pray for my sobriety, and Margo's sobriety, and everybody's sobriety under the sun. I explained to her not to do that, to, instead, pray for God's will for us. Here I am, hardly having any contact with this thing called God, explaining to a woman who's been in a nunnery for thirty years how to pray!

Eventually our contact [with Sister Anna Marie] dwindled, but we did hear that the nuns took new names—her new name was Sister Eustace—and that she was instrumental in opening a recovery house for women alcoholics, the first on the Peninsula, as far as I know. I understand that on her prayer list at that time, she had Pat's name as number one, and my name as number two. Pat died sober, and I'm still sober. So perhaps that's all a part of it.

In July, Pat and I bought a house that we couldn't afford and we asked Ginny and Margo if they'd like to rent the downstairs, and we moved in together. So this was the AA community for us, the four of us, and we were all sober, and very touchy about everything. There were a lot of things we didn't want to say in front of each other, somehow. So every night, we'd go to four different AA meetings, and then we'd come home and have coffee, or ice cream, and tell each other what we'd found out.

We were all trying to grab as much information we could. . . . We were also looking for any other lesbians we could spot. "Did you see anybody?" we'd ask each other. "No, did you?" We did spot one other woman, but she moved away before we could make contact. Other than [her], I don't know of any other gay people. We just didn't have them. I heard that some gay people went to the Telegraph Hill Group, and I went to see if I could find anybody, but if there was anyone there who was gay or lesbian, I didn't recognize them.

There was no gay AA going on that we knew about, until 1976 when Living Sober started. We went [to Living Sober] to see what was going on, and we were pretty sure it was a conflict of interest. The conflict was that AA didn't want special interest groups, like AA groups for doctors, where only doctors could go, instead of having meetings open to all alcoholics. We'd been sober quite a while, making it in straight AA, and our concern was that this was a branch-out into a dead end of some sort. So we certainly didn't go to any of those first conferences.

Since then I have quite changed my mind because, my heavens, gay people can find sobriety! I think it's due to the fact that they can go where they're safe about their gayness. I had a friend who looked very butch. She went to AA but she was so awfully uncomfortable that she just couldn't make it in straight AA.

We got a little seven-acre ranch in Sebastopol [in Sonoma County, California], and a couple of gay women we knew wanted to start a rap session [for lesbian alcoholics]. Pat said they ought to do an AA meeting. So they got one going, and Pat decided to go. I didn't go because I was being very anonymous. It was still illegal to be homosexual in California, and, immediately, my teaching credential would have been gone.

"My god, Ruth," Pat said when she came home that night. "There were eleven brand-new women there!" So from there on, we went to that meeting. That little group, the Stein Group, is still going. . . .

When I was a young woman, and got into the gay life, when I first got to the gay bars in San Francisco, I noticed right away that there were no old people around; there were no old lesbians. And one of the things that came up rather quickly was the number of lesbians in their thirties who committed suicide. The general idea was that being a lesbian was so bad that we destroyed ourselves. I believe that many of those suicides were alcoholics—alcoholics who had no way out. Without AA, I would have fit that category. So this is a great thing.

Now I live in Desert Hot Springs [in California]. There is a place in Palm Springs [called Sunny Dunes] where there are gay meetings every day. It's marvelous! Not that I have anything against straight AA, but this is so warm and loving. It's great. There's a lot of long-term sobriety too. Twenty years is nothing here.

[My partner,] Shawn, is inclined to hold my arm, as we walk down the street, and for the first time in my life, I feel okay about walking down the street and holding hands. If we are in Sunny Dunes, . . . and we feel like it, we can kiss. The atmosphere is entirely different from anything I've ever experienced. That freedom idea is really here.

George D.

[George attended his first AA meeting in Los Angeles in 1955. He and his partner live in New York City.]

My first couple of go-rounds in AA, I did not really have much to do with gay people. My non-AA social life was all gay, but initially, there was no gay social life for me in AA.

There were probably a lot of gay people like me, but—this was a long time ago—the ones who were more obvious—We used to have a saying in Chicago, "not for street wear." Have you ever heard that expression? The more flamboyant gay guys were great socially. We loved them. They were all lots of fun, and grist for a lot of great stories, but you really didn't want to be seen in public with them.

I had my last drink in 1961, and when I came back [to AA], my attitude was a little different. I met gay people I could relate to a little better, and when I moved to San Francisco, it was even more fun. There were more of us, and we were more integrated in San Francisco [AA]; the groups seemed more sophisticated; straight people were more sophisticated.

A friend of mine had . . . AA parties that were totally mixed. There wasn't any overt prejudice of any kind. All the straight people knew who the gay people were, but nobody ever talked about it. Of course, when the gay groups got going a lot of that died. Some of the straight people in San Francisco AA said that the gay meetings had ruined the straight meetings, that they weren't any fun anymore!

When a gay person spoke at those mixed meetings, did he say he was gay?

It was very rare for gay people to mention that they were gay in the course of a meeting, very rare. Those [who did were seen] as doing it out of anger, or exhibitionism. But *socially* they did, yes. Then the gay stuff would be pretty much out on the table.

In 1965, a friend of mine decided to throw the first big gay AA party. . . . [We] worked on the guest list and tried to dig up everybody who we knew was gay; we even invited two or three guys we weren't quite sure about! Everybody was pretty shocked when they all arrived at the party. They all looked at each other and said, "God, I didn't know *you* were gay!" . . .

The Gratitude Group in Sausalito was probably 50 percent gay [men] sometimes; the Telegraph Hill Group and the Under Thirty-Five Group in North Beach were both at least half gay [men].

So there was an "unacknowledged acknowledgment"?

You have to look at this within the context of the times. A man in the church I belong to here in New York died recently. . . . He was world famous, in fabrics and decorating. He left a large estate, and he'd earned it all himself. He'd had a remarkable life, but, even in his old age, he didn't—he was a product of a different era. . . . When you were around straight people it wasn't necessary to discuss gay things, although I think he changed a little bit because some of the women at the church talked about the hilarious stories he used to tell about his life in the Hamptons.

Look. He had a partner. He was extremely successful. He was rich as hell. He had this big apartment on Park Avenue, they'd been living together for years, everybody knew they were partners, but you didn't *talk* about this! It wasn't necessary to talk about this. That's the way gay guys were! And they were moving in extremely sophisticated circles, so everybody knows what's going on. They know how to handle it, and they're comfortable with it, and everybody plays by the same rules. . . .

When the gay meetings started, I went along, with mixed feelings about it. My closest gay friends were appalled by the idea and never got near the gay meetings, and they were plenty gay! We did not foresee that gay AA would get so big that guys would come in and never go anywhere else. There was a period when I was very troubled by that. I even wondered whether gay groups were a good idea. I don't know that we would have done anything different. I suppose it would have started anyway. But that was not a result we intended, and I was very unhappy about it for a long time. . . .

Would you tell me about your involvement with the first Living Sober conference?

Certainly. In 1975, the first year I was a delegate [to the General Service Conference], I got a letter from a member of the General Service Office [GSO] staff named Cora Louise. Enclosed was a letter they had received from this group that wanted to put on Living Sober, and an outrageous flier. The letter said what they were proposing to do, this thing that had never been done before, and that they wanted to do it in accord[ance with AA Traditions]. [As the area delegate,] Cora Louise asked me to contact these people who wanted help.

When I met with this group, I found didn't know any of them. They were all guys from the Haight-Ashbury area, with not much sobriety. There were many gay AAs around San Francisco at that time with solid, long-term sobriety, and none of them were involved. So you had this bunch of—well, you know the era—Haight-Ashbury types.

We talked about the flier. I said the tradition was to avoid getting AA into politics. That flier was so wonderful. It said something like, "Come march in the Gay Pride Parade!"

"Let's face it," I told them, "gay liberation is a political issue. If you raise it, you won't be in a very good position to object if the right-wingers in the Bible Belt and the conservative Christians in AA—and we've got them, just like they have us—come back and raise homophobia as a political issue."

After our second meeting, I began to see that the problems they were having didn't arise because they were gay. It was because they were alcoholics without a lot of sobriety. A straight group could be doing the same silly things. *[Laughing]* And they caught on very quickly. It's amazing how quickly they came around! Then they became Traditions lawyers. They were going to have a garage sale to raise money. One guy's mother was very excited about it, and wanted to donate a bunch of stuff. They argued for *two hours* about whether or not this violated the Seventh Tradition. Give me a break! I tried to tell them it wasn't a big deal.

Their next flier was almost prim and proper. When I showed it to Cora Louise, who came from a very aristocratic, old Southern family, she said *[mimicking her Southern accent]*, "Why, this is as decorous as an invitation to a coming-out party in Greenville, Mississippi."

I learned recently that the AA pamphlet A Member's Eye View of Alcoholics Anonymous *was written by a gay man named Alan McG. I understand Alan was a friend of yours. Can you tell me anything about him, and that wonderful pamphlet?*

Alan was probably the most articulate person I've ever met. He was an advertising genius, and a great writer. *A Member's Eye View* is a talk he was asked to give at the University of Southern California. His boss, who was an AA trustee, submitted it to the General Service Office. There was a lot of discussion about whether or not to publish it. Other than Bill Wilson's own writings, it's the only AA pamphlet that is such a personal statement. If you compare it to [AA's] other pamphlets, . . . this is "Alan's eye view" of AA.

Alan had never been to a gay group, so I took him to Fell Street once. It was small at the time, and we went around the table. Everyone talked about how wonderful it was to have a gay meeting, where you don't have to worry about being rejected. When it was his turn, Alan said, "Ah, I think I see what's going on now. The Indians are out there, and they're going to get us! We'll circle the wagons and hold out as long as we can!"

"I hear you guys talking about rejection," he said. "In my life, I have received a great deal of rejection from straight people, but nothing compared to the rejection I've received from gay people." That has been true in my life, too.

There is an outrageous story about the Fell Street Group. . . . At the time, Alfred Kinsey was doing a study on gay people. One of his guys was looking at gay sexuality and alcoholism, and, one night, someone brought the Kinsey man to the meeting.

There were eight to ten of us there, in that same room, on Fell Street. We were all being very prim and proper, *very* dignified, for the Kinsey man, when all of a sudden, there is a big commotion at the door, lots of noise and crashing, and, finally, Chuck O. comes staggering in, roaring drunk.

Everyone falls completely silent.

Chuck slowly manages to pull himself up, and then he starts sliding along the wall. "Girllls," he sayd, "yer mmother's drunnk." So much for our efforts to be dignified for the Kinsey guy!

I don't know what other history you've gotten, but I can assure you that, in the beginning, [the Fell Street] Group split the gay AA community in San Francisco. Friendships were strained. A lot of our close friends wouldn't have anything to do with it. They thought it was terrible. They were concerned that there was no need, which was probably true, in San Francisco because so many of the groups were heavily if not predominantly gay. They were concerned that it was divisive. And there was a lot of fear.

I was not an enthusiastic supporter. But I went along with it. I was one of the first secretaries, and we were so nervous that [the Fell Street Group] elected five secretaries—one for each week of the month, [and] a fifth, in case there was an extra Friday. We wanted to distribute the responsibility, so that whatever wrath there was within the fellowship couldn't all come down on one person.

Living Sober's Infamous First Flier

The first Living Sober conference was held in June 1976 and was attended by about 200 people. Attendance grew rapidly in the decades that followed, peaking in the early 1990s at over 5,000. Today, attendance averages around 2000.

"Roundups," as conferences hosted by the gay, lesbian, bisexual, and transgendered members of AA and Al-Anon are widely known, are now held in cities all over the United States, and in cities outside the United States as well. At last count there were over fifty cities with an annual gathering.

Living Sober's first flier, in keeping with the theme of the bicentennial year, was designed to look like an American flag. The words, "SAY IT LOUD! LIVING SOBER, GAY & PROUD!" were repeated over and over around the perimeter, in bold letters half an inch high. This eye-catching banner framed the following announcement:

SAY IT LOUD! LIVING SOBER, GAY & PROUD!

Gay Alcoholics Anonymous with Gay Al-Anon of San Francisco invites all GAA and Alcoholics Together members in the Western United States to join in a 1976 Western Regional Round-Up on Friday, Saturday, and Sunday of June 25, 26, and 27.

June 25-27 is the weekend of San Francisco's Gay Pride Week. Neither AA nor any special interest group within AA endorses outside issues or causes. This Regional Round-Up will NOT be listed as one of the groups publicly supporting Gay Pride Week, nor will it be listed as part of the activities of the week, but for those who are now able to enjoy the gay life through sobriety, Gay Pride Week is particularly significant. AA has made possible a new way of life—a program of sharing. That's what this conference is all about: sharing at the individual and group level.

To the best of our knowledge, the concept of Gay Alcoholics Anonymous began in San Francisco and we will have the opportunity of hearing one of the founders speak. Depending on resources received, a variety of structures could occur (i.e., workshops, mini-marathons, women's groups, stag groups, films, rap sessions, etc.). Should response be minimal we would have, at least, one huge meeting wrapped up with a rock band boogie.

We NEED to hear from groups as soon as possible in order to set up the structure for those interested; we can either arrange "package deals" with hotels or space in private homes. Child care will be available. But all this needs to be arranged long in advance. Please read this announcement to your group(s) and inquire about interest in participation.

We look forward to a naturally high weekend
to be shared with those of us within Alcoholics Anonymous.

****

PLEASE RESPOND RAPIDLY!

Don Hiemforth, Coordinator
402 Duboce Avenue, San Francisco, California 94117
(415) 431-4708 (please, no collect calls)

****

****

Registration will include:
DYNAMITE BOOGIE BANDS
A FLOOR SHOW
PLUS
Some Unbelievable Surprises

****

Send Registration Fee of $3.00 directly to:
Don Hiemforth
402 Duboce Avenue, San Francisco, California 94117
(415) 431-4708

Extra contributions are needed as expenses mount.
If you can contribute above the call—GREAT!

****

GAA: ___AT: ___Gay Al-Anon: ___
Name: _____
Address: _____
City: _____
Zip (required): _____

****

"The service we render to others is really the rent we pay
for our room on this earth."

****

Moss B.

[Moss got sober in 1975.]

In 1969 I moved to San Francisco and started school at the San Francisco Art Institute. At the Art Institute, you could smoke dope in class. We weren't supposed to, but nobody really cared if you did. So it was freewheeling, anything goes, Student Power, 1969, in San Francisco. It was fabulous.

. . . I met a woman from Chile, who was hitchhiking around the United States. This was during the time of Allende.

"You should come to Chile," she said. "There are bags of marijuana, plates of cocaine, and the best wine in the world for less than a dollar a bottle." I got a student loan, and bought a one-way plane ticket to Chile.

We got married in Chile. The thinking was, *People should be bisexual. This is really how everybody in the world is. Everybody should just be able to get along with everybody.*

Well, this may have worked for a few people, back in enlightened San Francisco, but it certainly didn't work in Chile. . . . We came back to San Francisco in 1971. I recall going right to a party at the Art Institute and that I was wearing a long leather coat, platform shoes, a Panama hat, and that we were snorting coke using $100 bills. We thought, "Oh, we have *arrived!*" She and I split up not long after that because, well, because I'm gay. But we stayed married a number of years so that she could get her green card.

I was twenty-one when we got back, and could go to the bars. The Capri in North Beach was the bar after the Black Cat, and we could dance at the Capri. Pat Bond was the bouncer at the Capri.[3] Pat would stand at the door, and if a police car came by she'd shine a light on the back of the bar. The bartender would turn up the lights, the police would walk through, and we'd all be standing there. Then the police would leave, and that would be it. When I got back from Chile there were a few Polk Street bars, the big disco bars, [and] the Stud was there, south of Market.

[On the second anniversary of Stonewall, 1971], there was a police raid on the Stud. [At] closing time there were eight to ten police cars out front and a paddy wagon. The police had blocked off the street at either end, and a man was trying to get out of the alley in his car. I saw a cop drop to the ground and yell, "My god, this guy hit me!" But I don't think the guy hit him with his car. I was standing right there. The man in the car panicked. He sped off into the street, but it was blocked. So he got out of his car, and ran past us down the alley. Then the police started firing—past this whole crowd of people. We had to dive under the parked cars to try to be safe! They didn't care who they hurt.

I got picked up for drunk driving and I went to an AA meeting in San Francisco. I arrived late, and . . . . people were talking about "Steps" and "character defects." I thought the whole thing was very quaint. Then this mad queen starts talking about how lust is a character defect, and how God was going to remove lust from my heart.

What in God's name is going on here? I thought. *I love lust! I can't stand God. This is obviously not the group for me.* Finally, the meeting ended, and I fled. All these people tried to give me their phone numbers. I just grabbed them, and then I threw them away.

At my third AA meeting I heard Lorraine C. speak. Lorraine lived in Tiburon, or Sausalito. She was very well quaffed. Her hair was done up, and she was dripping in gold jewelry. I was late for the meeting again, so I had to sit in the first row. Lorraine told her whole story right to me—about having to crawl to the refrigerator to get her booze, about [being] strung out on ups [amphetamines] and downs [barbiturates] and booze, all at the same time. Her story was absolutely incredible. She was telling me Zen koans.

When she finished, she called on me. I said something about how [the people in AA] have been there the whole time [I was drinking]. Then she talked about a gold thread. She said that there was a gold thread between us, and I could feel the gold thread. That was the magic I experienced that evening. I was very lucky to have that immediate connection; some people never do.

Lorraine put me in touch with Bud C., who became my sponsor. Bud and I became real close. I would never have had the guts to go up to someone like Bud, who had eighteen years [of] sobriety. But Lorraine made me do it!

I understand you helped organize Living Sober, in 1976. Would you tell me about that experience?

There were a bunch of people on the planning committee who had just slightly more time sober than I did. We were all ex-hippies. Actually, we were all *still* hippies. Lewis D. and Don H. were the mad queens who kind of got the thing going. It was almost a political statement—part of Gay Power. The parades were starting to get huge then.[4] It was an outgrowth of the Gay Movement in San Francisco.

The idea was to put on a world conference. San Francisco would host it the first year. Then another city would host it the next, and so on. The committee meetings were total madness because none of us had any concept of the AA Traditions. We were trying to get free coffee, free space, free money, and free everything. And we could have gotten it, but Bob H., who knew a bit more about the Traditions than we did, started saying things like, "Well, no. You're not supposed to do that."

"You've got to be out of your mind!" we all told him, because we had no money, zero. Then somebody donated some money, so there was a little nest egg for printing. To this day, I don't know who [it was].[5]

A lot of the old queens who'd been sober for a while were tsk-tsking the whole thing. They were horrified that we were doing this because we were violating the Traditions, because we were sending out all these fliers. They thought we should all just blend in, and not draw attention to ourselves. "It's nice to have a couple of gay meetings," they said. "But, *really,* why do we need this?" Then they said, "Well, *we* certainly aren't going to come!"

But Bud C. said he would come. Then a bunch of people who were starting recovery places [for gay alcoholics], like Henry Olaff House and Acceptance House, said they would come. Then a few more said they would come, and that's when George D. got involved.

The steering committee had sent a letter to the General Service Office in New York, with a conference flier that was just outrageous. You can see why the people in New York were horrified. It said things like "Gay Power!" and "Power to the People!" and "Sobriety will help us in our fight for gay equality in the world!"

George was the Bay Area delegate to the General Service Conference. When New York received our flier they called him and said, "Would you please go check out these people? They are out of control!" Which we were. We just didn't know how to do a conference.

So George came to our steering committee meeting. He told us there were certain things we couldn't do because of AA Traditions.

"Okay," he said, "listen up. Here is the packet from the World Service Office that tells you how to start a conference. Read it. Yes, I know it would be nice to get free coffee—"

"But it's already been donated!" we said.

"Yes, but you can't accept it because we don't do that." He had to really walk us through this thing.

"Promise me you won't mail out any more fliers until I've okay'd them," he said. "If you do that, I'll attend the conference." So George gave us the kiss of approval. The big thing was whether we would be [listed] in the [conference calendar in the] *AA Grapevine.* In May, the announcement for Living Sober appeared in the *Grapevine* calendar, and the conference was on.[6]

I had to chair the big meeting Saturday night and introduce the speaker, and I was nervous as hell. My stutter came back pretty badly, when I was newly sober, and I obsessed about what might happen. Would I get totally get tongue-tied? Would I pass out? Would I throw up? What happened was that my legs started shaking, and I hadn't imagined that. So I just noted it and went on, and I got through it.

In our view, the conference was a total success. We didn't know if anybody would show up at all because all these old queens were just trashing us, right and left— *[Laughing]* Actually, I shouldn't say "old queens"; they weren't nearly as old as I am now! Some of the criticism was certainly warranted. We had violated major AA Traditions. But then we were reigned in. George said, "Okay, here's how you do a conference," and AA worked. Everybody was just horrified by what we were doing. It was great.

Can you tell me any more about the men you knew who got sober before the gay groups started?

There was always a huge gay contingent at the downtown St. Mary's meetings, probably fifty out of 200 to 300 people on a given night. Afterward, we'd go to Miz Brown's on Polk Street. These queens would sit and dish, and I would sit there with my mouth open, enraptured by this gossip. They came from a whole different tradition—the Empress Balls [events organized by José Sarria, from the Black Cat, and other members of San Francisco's drag community]. There was a whole slew of them from that era, and long-term sobriety in that group. There was one old queen who'd gotten Twelve-Stepped by Bill Wilson. That was his claim to fame! He lived in the Tenderloin and helped a lot of people get sober.

Of the thirteen people on the original Living Sober steering committee, I think I am the only one left. Everyone else has died, either of old age, or AIDS . . . No, AIDS. *[He stops.]*

I got involved in Al-Anon, through Bud, because I kept falling in love with all these alcoholics. After five years, I met someone. We were together thirteen years. We bought a house. *[He falls silent.]*

Now I'm on retreat from the world here, in Florida. I fled the Bay Area—all the death and dying, all the loss. I think I'm starting to come out of that now.

Last weekend I shared at a meeting about long-term sobriety. If you don't die, I said, and you keep going to meetings, you get long-term sobriety. You get a life. But you also get history. You become part of the story—The Story, with a capital T and a capital S!

There's another Living Sober conference people still talk about, the one in 1980, at Fort Mason.[7] We decorated that huge pier building with trees, and all this diaphanous material. I helped put it up. We called it "Swag Heaven." There's a story about two men who came to Living Sober in 1980, who'd been members of regular AA for years, but had never been to a gay conference before. They walked into the meeting hall [and saw] all that white material, [gently] billowing in the breeze, and thought it was the most beautiful sight they'd ever seen.

They looked at each other and said, "This must be what heaven is like."

Brenda C.

[Brenda C. shared this story about her first conference.]

My first Living Sober was in 1978. I was in my first thirty days of sobriety, and I had no idea what it was, but I'd told my friend I'd meet her there, so I went.

It was at the Unitarian church, and as I'm walking up the front steps, I'm thinking, *What am I doing this for? I'm not an alcoholic.*

At the front door, I think, *I'm not a lesbian! No, I don't need to do this,* and I turn to leave. And as I'm walking down the stairs, this big, nellie queen bursts out the door and comes running after me, arms flailing in the air. She grabs my hand and says, "Welcome! Welcome to Living Sober! Come in! Come in!" and we go inside.

I kept thinking, *What am I doing here? I'm not an alcoholic! Who* are *these people, anyway? What the hell is going on?*

It was a pretty small gathering, but I stayed. At one point in the meeting, they asked everyone with less than thirty days of sobriety to stand up, and everybody clapped for us. I thought it was a trick. I'd heard you weren't supposed to get involved with newcomers. I thought they made us stand up so everyone would know who not to have an affair with. I was angry because I really wanted to have an affair!

They served doughnuts, as a snack. I was trying to be healthy, and I told them they ought to serve fruit instead.

"If you want to change something," they told me, "you have to go down to General Planning. You have to work on the next conference."

So I went down there. I told them they should serve fruit, so my first job at Living Sober was heading up the new fruit committee.

I had a love affair with Living Sober. Going to Living Sober was just something everybody did. You were expected to go, and to drag along newcomers, if you could, the same way I was dragged. "Okay," we'd say, "I'll pick you up, and we'll go!"

Chapter 13

AA's Pamphlet
for Lesbian and Gay Alcoholics

At any given point in time AA's literature spells out what AA is—its culture. The literature is the reference point, both for affirming AA's consensus about itself and for dealing with the pressures of change. It is no accident that every [AA General Service] Conference devotes the greatest proportion of its discussions to AA's written word.

Joan Jackson
AA [nonalcoholic] Trustee, 1983-1992

Introduction

This is the story of AA's pamphlet for lesbian and gay alcoholics. It is also the story of how AA literature is made.

Since its first printing in 1939, *Alcoholics Anonymous,* AA's "Big Book," has sold more than twenty-one million copies. At last count, it had been translated into forty-three different languages, in addition to English (Big Book Facts 2001). *Twelve Steps and Twelve Traditions* has been translated into thirty different languages. In addition to these and other books, AA also publishes scores of meeting materials and pamphlets, as well as publications for physicians, clergy members, and law enforcement personnel.

AA's Ninth Tradition states, "AA, as such, ought never be organized; but we may create service boards or committees directly responsible to those they serve." That's a lot of publishing for an organization

The History of Gay People in Alcoholics Anonymous
Published by The Haworth Press, Inc., 2007. All rights reserved.
doi:10.1300/5699_13

that "ought never be organized." Who, exactly, is in charge of all this publishing?

AA's General Service Conference

Decisions regarding AA's literature, and all other matters concerning Alcoholics Anonymous as a whole, are formulated and expressed through the collective voice of the organization's annual General Service Conference. The General Service Conference (GSC) convenes in New York each April for seven days and is attended by approximately 400 people from across the United States and Canada.

Elected by their fellow AAs to represent them, conference delegates serve a two-year term. Delegates participate on one of eleven standing conference committees. For example, the Literature Committee addresses issues submitted to the conference related to AA literature.[1] Conference decisions, called "Advisory Actions," are not mandates, but recommendations that AA's members, service boards, and committees are encouraged to adopt.

Literature for Minority Groups in AA

AA's literature plays an important role in the organization's outreach to the alcoholic who still suffers. For example, the pamphlet *Do You Think You're Different?* contains stories from AA members who are old, young, lesbian, gay, atheist, agnostic, black, Native American, Jewish, and famous, as well as clergy members and "low-bottom" and "high-bottom" alcoholics (Alcoholics Anonymous 2000; A Benediction from Bill 1952). Table 13.1 lists the names and publication dates of AA's pamphlets for some of its minority members.

Decision Making and Unanimity at the General Service Conference

After five intensive days in workshops and committee meetings, everyone assembles in the main hall. That time is dedicated to a series of general sessions dedicated to committee reports, recommendations, and decision making. Great care is taken at these voting ses-

TABLE 13.1. AA Publications for Minorities, 1956-1999

Year	Publication (Pamphlet)
1952	*A.A. for the Woman*
1969	*Young People and A.A.*
1976	*Do You Think You're Different?*
1979	*Time to Start Living: Stories of Those Who Came to A.A. in Their Later Years*
1989	*A.A. and the Gay/Lesbian Alcoholic; A.A. for the Native North American*
2001	*Can A.A. Help Me Too? Black/African Americans Share Their Stories*

sions to thoroughly discuss the issues presented, so that conference decisions are reached by unanimous vote. Decisions made this way are said to have been made with complete "unanimity." But what happens when unanimity cannot be reached at the conference? When opinion remains strongly divided?

After the recommendations of each committee are presented, voting members of the conference are invited to share comments using the microphones on the assembly hall floor. If the issue under consideration is controversial, lines will begin to form behind the microphones, as people wait to speak. And if those lines remain long, other agenda items will be put aside to enable the discussion to continue. If it becomes clear that unanimity cannot be reached, the conference will often postpone making a decision until the following year. And as a result, the more divided the conference is on a particular issue, the longer it will take to reach a decision. This is what happened when the issue under discussion was an AA pamphlet for gay alcoholics.

Following decisions reached with anything less than complete unanimity, members of the conference whose votes did not carry, known as those in the minority, are invited to speak. Describing the importance of the voice of the minority in *Twelve Concepts for World Service,* Bill Wilson writes:

[A]ll minorities—whether in our staffs, committees, corporate boards, or among the Trustees—should be encouraged to file minority reports whenever they feel a majority to be in considerable error. And when a minority considers an issue to be such a grave one that a mistaken decision could seriously affect AA as

a whole, it should then charge itself with the actual duty of presenting a minority report to the Conference.
. . . [W]e recognize that minorities frequently can be right; that even when they are partly or wholly in error they still perform a most valuable service when, by asserting their "Right of Appeal," they compel a thorough-going debate on important issues. The well-heard minority, therefore, is our chief protection against an uninformed, misinformed, hasty, or angry majority. (Alcoholics Anonymous 2001, p. 22)

Table 13.2 lists the conference's decisions regarding a pamphlet for homosexual alcoholics in the years between 1981 and 1989 (Alcoholics Anonymous 2000).

Should AA Publish a Pamphlet for Homosexuals?

In a 1992 interview with Nancy T., a 1981/1982 conference delegate who served on the Literature Committee, D. R., recalled the dis-

TABLE 13.2. Conference Actions Regarding a Pamphlet for Gay Alcoholics

Year	Advisory Action
1981	That: "The suggestion to publish a pamphlet for the homosexual alcoholic be tabled until the 1982 Conference to allow time for all delegates to get the group conscience from the groups in their areas." And that: ". . . [A] pamphlet for the homosexual alcoholic be placed on the 1982 Conference Literature Committee agenda."
1982	"A draft of a pamphlet be developed for the homosexual alcoholic to be considered by the next year's Conference."
1983	"The 1983 draft of the pamphlet for the homosexual alcoholic be approved for circulation" . . . so that next year we can decide "whether or not the fellowship will publish and distribute a pamphlet for the homosexual alcoholic."
1984	"The draft of a pamphlet for the homosexual alcoholic be dropped." And that: The Conference ". . . not develop a pamphlet for the homosexual alcoholic, as the need is currently addressed in the pamphlet, *Do You Think You're Different?*"
1988	"A draft of a pamphlet for the gay/lesbian alcoholic be prepared and reviewed by the 1989 Conference."
1989	"The manuscript for a pamphlet for gay/lesbian alcoholics be approved . . . and that the title be *A.A. and the Gay/Lesbian Alcoholic.*"

cussions about an AA pamphlet for gay alcoholics. D. R. was a first-year delegate on the Literature Committee when the request for a pamphlet first appeared on their agenda.

Reading the correspondence that came in to the General Service Office staff on the subject of a gay pamphlet—and there was a tremendous amount of correspondence which was given [to] us—members of the Literature Committee and I went through all the letters, and I was astounded at the number of people that had written in. . . . I saw a transition. From the time the subject was first brought up in a Virginia assembly, when it was just almost either taboo or a joke, as far as they were concerned, to becoming a very serious matter and being considered.

I think it was because many people working in service on the district level have encountered the same thing we do in our Intergroup's answering services: we need something [to give people calling us for help]. We can tell people that we do understand that there are gay groups and lesbian groups, that everyone is welcome, it's open, but when you have a written pamphlet it gives [your assurances] a validity that the spoken word does not give.

In 1982, following the conference's request for a draft, a committee comprised of members of the General Service Office (GSO) staff and the newly formed International Advisory Council of Homosexual Men and Women in Alcoholics Anonymous convened to prepare one. The group produced three versions of the pamphlet over a six-month period. Each was reviewed by the members of the GSO staff and the trustees' Literature Committee, and in the spring of 1983 the final draft was submitted to the conference for review. But even at the committee's final meeting, there were concerns about what they'd produced. Nancy T. recalled:

It was like a tiny little Big Book; that was our working vision of it. [The] draft was felt by all of us to be somewhat too Gay Lib–oriented, but we went forward with it. We had quite a number of stories, but some of them were felt to be controversial. We had one from a gay Roman Catholic priest. We had one from a drag queen. These are elements within the gay community we know and accept, and it's no big deal, but within the larger AA community, they were felt to be extremely controversial. So we picked some vanilla-type people to be our stories, in the back of this pamphlet, and we proceeded with this.

Lois F. was GSO staff member for many years, and one of the conference coordinators in the early 1980s. She recalled some of the conferences where the pamphlet was discussed:

> I definitely saw a need for [a gay pamphlet], and spoke strongly in favor, though it was turned down, which was very disappointing to me. Some of the delegates were against it because they thought we were getting involved in outside issues.
>
> At one point, a man in the office who wasn't gay, but who was very sympathetic to gays, got involved with the project. He hired a gay writer, but the writer was kind of an advocate. His writing style was militant, and if you read between the lines, it just didn't read like AA literature usually reads. I think the tone of the pamphlet was one of the things that did it in at the conference.[2]

In 1987, three years after the 1984 decision to drop the 1983 draft, a member of the AA trustees' Literature Committee invited a senior member of the *AA Grapevine* staff, named Ames S., to draft a new version. Ames spoke with me about his experience working on the pamphlet:

> I'd heard stories about how long and how vehemently this pamphlet had been rejected over the years. Yet, when I entered into the process, everything went extremely smoothly.
>
> As I see it, the pamphlet is less about being gay or lesbian, and more about getting into and understanding recovery. What was exciting to me was being able to take the experience of a particular culture and translate that into AA language so that readers could see beyond the components of being gay, or lesbian, to the fact that they were alcoholic. One's sexual orientation, one's race, one's education level, one's status with the federal government, such as whether you're a former convict, all of that really is secondary in AA.

All of the prejudices, the painful stuff we go through in society at large, are reflected in the rooms of AA. There is racism. There is gender bias. There's all that stuff, without a doubt, but the proportions are considerably smaller. It's always incredible to me that it really is the exception, not the rule.

I've always had the feeling that [the conference's decision to publish a pamphlet for gay alcoholics] was a moment where the fellowship as a whole moved beyond its prejudices and limitations. And I found that to be true for me on a personal level, as a straight man working on a pamphlet for gay and lesbian alcoholics. It was both a challenge, and gave me a sense of meaning and of pride, if you will. When I walk into a meeting and see that pamphlet there, I am glad I was able to participate in that way.

A number of years ago an article by a former AA trustee named Joan Jackson appeared in the *Grapevine*. One of Joan's theories about AA literature was that once a pamphlet was produced on a particular topic, it is almost as if the problem it was produced to address disappears. That in the chewing-over process that inaugurates the pamphlets, the social problems and concerns are often worked out, so that by the time the pamphlet arrives, it's almost not a problem anymore.

Sometimes What We're Searching for Finds Us

I searched high and low for Joan Jackson's article, after talking with Ames. I combed through *Grapevine* collections and indexes in the San Francisco Central Office and the Northern Coastal Area Archives, to no avail, and I gave up. Then, nearly a year later, I found an assortment of old *Grapevine*s in my mother-in-law's basement and grabbed a handful to read. They sat on the desk in my office for six months. Then they sat on my bedside table for six more. One night, when I couldn't sleep, I remembered the *Grapevine*s and decided to read awhile. Reaching over in the dark, I grabbed an issue from the top of the stack, and turned on the light. Opening it to a page at random, I nearly fell out of bed, for there was Joan Jackson. She was peering out from a small black-and-white photograph above an article titled "Communication and Culture." Sometimes what we're searching for finds us.

Dr. Jackson served as a Class A (nonalcoholic) trustee on the AA General Service Board from 1983 to 1992. She held a doctorate in sociology and was Alcoholics Anonymous's first woman trustee. The article Ames told me about appeared in the *Grapevine* shortly after Joan retired as an AA trustee, and it catalyzed my understanding of how AA literature is made.

> . . . One of the issues which has been of intense and mounting concern since I first attended the [General Service] Conference is the question of who shall be accepted as a member of AA.
>
> It seems to me that this problem of who can be helped by AA has always been with us. It was there, but less acute, in 1951. At that time, the . . . probability that a newcomer would want to discuss anything which members would experience as not relevant was almost zero. . . . Most AA members had been through the same things. Identification was instant and thus so was helpfulness.
>
> However, even then, "strangers" were appearing. Some younger people sought help, and doubts were expressed about whether they could be helped before they "were ready." Women arrived, and there were after-meeting complaints about inability to identify with their problems. It now seems very hard to imagine that the young and women really caused problems for groups at one time since both now have been embraced by AA. Over the years, other new kinds of alcoholics sought help, were briefly seen as problems, and then were absorbed into the Fellowship.
>
> . . . [T]ime and again, AA has been faced with answering the calls for help from alcoholics who pose problems AA has not coped with before. Often the AA response has been to create a pamphlet for that particular type of alcoholic. In the discussion about the need for such a pamphlet, AA has identified what the problems of such people are in "working the program." In writing the pamphlets and then in using them, AA members and the newcomers have acquired greater understanding. And gradually, mutual problems disappear and the newcomer is absorbed into AA. As a nonalcoholic observer, it has seemed to me that, once such a pamphlet appears, the subject of that particular kind of problem and newcomer does not come up at subsequent Conferences. Creation of a pamphlet is a sign of an unresolved problem; elimination of a pamphlet points to a problem which has been solved. (Jackson 1993)

AA literature develops slowly over time, guided by the collective effort of the General Service Conference. Although the issue of a pamphlet for gay and lesbian alcoholics was controversial from the start, in the end, the members of the conference recognized its importance and brought it to fruition.

Jackson writes, "Creation of a pamphlet is a sign of an unresolved problem; elimination of a pamphlet points to a problem that has been solved." When alcoholics once thought of as different are no longer seen as different, a special piece of literature to welcome them into AA will no longer be needed. But as long as prejudice exists in our culture, pamphlets for AA's many minorities will stand guard in the literature rack, upholding AA's Third Tradition and keeping its doors open to all.

Chapter 14

The Home Front

Introduction

The people whose stories appear in this chapter entered AA in cities, towns, and hamlets far removed from cities with established gay communities, like those in Los Angeles, New York, and San Francisco. Many of them were the first openly gay people to attend AA meetings in the places where they lived.

Norma J.

[Norma got sober in Florida in 1976.]

I was teaching, in a job I'd been in for a long time, and one of my teaching buddies was a lesbian. She was an important teacher in the school system; she had a high place, and we were teaching in Dade County. She thought it was very important to be in hiding. . . . I was not drinking; she was. She was a lesbian; I thought I was straight. And I fell in love with her, though she didn't want me as a lover because she was a dear friend. She said, "Since you are in the process of coming out, I will introduce you to my friends." And she started inviting me to their homes because that's what they did on weekends; hiding lesbians partied at home.

I got to be close with that group of women. I heard my first coming-out stories at their parties. But pretty soon, I wasn't interested in hiding. I was reading *Lesbian Nation*,[1] and I got very excited because I identified with that book from beginning to end. I wanted to be *out!* . . .

The History of Gay People in Alcoholics Anonymous
Published by The Haworth Press, Inc., 2007. All rights reserved.
doi:10.1300/5699_14

I wanted to celebrate! I wasn't interested in hiding, and they weren't interested in me. An out lesbian wasn't any good in that group.

Once I came out, I was out with a vengeance. I was in the first available Gay Pride Parade. . . . I've always been an activist, and I was proud to be a lesbian right away. It was a very political time, too—that Anita Bryant time in south Florida.[2] . . . I felt threatened by the lesbians in the National Organization for Women, until I got sober. Once I was sober and out, I could be active in anything!

The first gay and lesbian AA meeting I ever went to was at the Metropolitan Community Church, in Fort Lauderdale, Florida, in an old house they'd converted into a church. There must have been forty men there, and me, and one other woman. I'd never felt at home with gay men, but somehow I felt at home in this meeting. People were very sociable and I felt included right away. When I was first coming out, I felt . . . heroic. I was a righteous, heroic activist! And being heroic, I loved being included. I loved the "attagirls" I got at that meeting, and of course I kept going, and I began to recover—not only through gay AA meetings, but also through women's AA meetings. I wasn't the only lesbian in those meetings, but I was the only lesbian who was out.

Soon we had a clubhouse in Fort Lauderdale for gay and lesbian recovering people, and I was a part of that, and soon we had a gay and lesbian Roundup in south Florida. So I was a very happy dyke. It was clear I was a political animal in recovery. So, by around 1979, when it came time to start the clubhouse, and the Roundup, there were a lot of political issues involved, and I was very much in the middle of it. It was an effort by the women in the group to include lesbians equally, no longer calling things "gay," but "gay and lesbian," no longer assuming that the "right people" would take leadership, but having a man and a woman as [committee] cochairs.

Not everyone agreed that feminist values were important, but it happened because we pushed for it: equal representation on planning committees, equal representation in leadership, and equal numbers of male and female speakers at our conference. Not in the club—there were many more men than women in the club, so there were many more male speakers at speaker meetings. But at the conference, there was equality. And I assume it's still that way, because we wrote it into the bylaws. At the clubhouse, we had a bylaw requirement that if we had a male chair one year, we'd have a female the next. We had to have those rules. If we hadn't, there would have rarely been a woman in leadership because there were so many more men in recovery in those days.[3]

I was part of the Fort Lauderdale Intergroup, but only briefly. . . . In those days, there were a lot of undercurrents . . . [like] people questioning the validity of our group. To my knowledge, nobody in AA ever did anything overt, but the undercurrents were there. There were undercurrents from some of the men about *women* participating in AA, even if those women were straight! But if our meetings weren't supported, they were acknowledged. And not many years later, they were supported. Intergroup referred people to our meetings, or they'd give them the phone number of someone they knew was gay or lesbian. Our Seventh Tradition donations were accepted and our meetings appeared in the directory.

I don't know how or why it happened, but some years after my partner Judy and I got together, I was in a dry drunk that lasted four years. I stopped going to meetings. I went back to compulsive overeating [Norma is also a member of Overeaters Anonymous]. I went back to blaming. I went back to manipulating, being right all the time, pushing other people around—all of it. I went back to every old way I had, except for drinking. Drinking just seemed too lethal. I was miserable. I guess I had to prove to myself that AA helps with life.

I left teaching, and Judy and I moved to San Miguel de Allende, a city . . . in the state of Guanajuato, in Mexico. There are roughly 5,000 English-speaking residents, many of whom live here year-round. In summer, teachers come to further their education in art, language, and music education, and art students come for a summer of work.

Judy and I used to go to Puerto Vallarta in the winter. They have wonderful recovery in Puerto Vallarta and, in spite of myself, I started going to meetings and loving it. [When we came] back from Puerto Vallarta . . . we started a women's meeting here. I'm active, and I sponsor a lot. We have a nucleus of about twenty-five people, and meetings every day. We rarely have a meeting here with only regulars. There's lots of vitality in these kinds of communities because visitors come and share their experience, strength, and hope.

Even though it's obvious I'm a dyke, . . . it is necessary for me to say so. I was forty-four when I came out to Norma, and I was the last one to know I was a lesbian. I'm always the last to know anything, so it's important to me to out myself.

I guess twenty-six years [of sobriety means I'm] probably an old-timer, but I know a lot of people who have as much sobriety as I do. What's constant is the fact that recovery continues to change as long as I am honest and open. I've always experienced the H.O.W. of the program backward. I get willing first, open second, and honest third. *[Laughing]* I think that's because denial is my middle name! But I know that's common in recovery. Long-term sobriety has shown me that I'm just one of the people on the bus. I'm not out there in a limo!

There used to be no time when I sat quietly. Today, there are lots of times I don't say anything at meetings. Sometimes I don't have much to offer, or other people are saying it. Long-term sobriety has given me the willingness to shut up and listen.

I recently [got] involved with a school here for troubled high school–aged kids, called the DeSisto School. Mostly they are troubled about alcohol, drugs, food, sex, and addictions. The students are not there voluntarily. Someone has put them there, and paid for it. So they don't go there willingly. They get willing through the process. It's all about kids discovering recovery. A few months ago, I proposed a course in mural making, and they took me up on it.

At the end of my teaching career, I was on a dry drunk and had some repair work to do. That's why I had to go back to teaching. *[Laughing]* Of course, I didn't know that when I volunteered to make the mural with the kids! What an opportunity.

It's painful sometimes, but now, in this wonderful therapeutic environment, I'm repairing the harm I've done in the past. Yesterday was a painful day, and I was grateful to have a meeting to go to where I could talk about it.

I don't experience long-term sobriety as different from short-term sobriety. I learn as much from newcomers as I do from old-timers, maybe more. The rawness helps. I try to let myself be open and raw when something's going on, to speak before I know how to say it nicely. Sometimes things come out while I'm talking, and the people at the meeting discover it with me. I try my damnedest, as soon as I know something, or even before, to talk about it. If I'm willing to blurt things out as they hit my heart, I get a whole lot more.

Doug H.

[Doug grew up in Pink Hill, North Carolina, a small town about 100 miles southeast of Raleigh. He has been sober since 1977.][1]

While attending the University of North Carolina in Chapel Hill, I was arrested for driving while intoxicated. My attorney suggested I go to the mental health clinic and there I was referred to Alcoholics Anonymous. Later that year I moved back to a place near my old hometown 120 miles east of Chapel Hill.

I attended some meetings there in a cement-block meeting house, on a dirt tobacco road, and I was the youngest. They were filled with smoke, and a lot of crude questions were posed to me, not about my homosexuality, because that was unknown, but painful questions, like, "Are you getting all the nookie you want these days?" Only they weren't saying "nookie."

How do you overcome the feeling of isolation—what the Big Book calls "the chilling vapor that is loneliness"? The AA program gave me tools to deal with that isolation. I taped a note to the dashboard of my car that said, "God will not let fear control my life today."

In 1978 I saw a little blurb in the calendar at the back of the *Grapevine* about Living Sober: "presented by the gay and lesbian members of AA in San Francisco." I had just come back from vacation. I'd driven all the way to Key West, Florida, and back again, but when I saw that announcement, I said, "I must go. These are my people. Of all the people in the universe, these are the ones!"

I wrote to the P.O. Box for a registration form and received a wonderful handwritten response from Tom H. . . . "I bet this is a lonely guy from North Carolina," he thought, "who saw our announcement in the *Grapevine*, who would really appreciate a handwritten note." And he was absolutely right. When I got his letter, I was jumping for joy. Tom later became my sponsor.

Living Sober was a turning point in my life. It was a pink cloud. It was beyond my wildest dreams. It was all the Promises coming true at the same time.[4] *There were other gay people in Alcoholics Anony-*

mous! After that, I became what we used to call a Roundup junkie, because going back to a small town in eastern North Carolina was very hard.

When I started going to Roundups, I began to learn self-acceptance. I used to be ashamed of where I came from. I come from down a dirt road, in a little place called Pink Hill, North Carolina. It was easy for me to love and accept others, but I had to learn to do that for myself. If others could love me for who I was, then I could do the same.

I thrived on Roundups, and the knowledge that they existed. The effort I made to get to them, and the experiences I had there, gave me the strength to go on. One of the things that impressed me was how I could meet total strangers and, by the time the weekend was over, we felt as though we'd known each other all our lives. . . . There's no feeling quite like connecting with another gay or lesbian member of AA. That's why gay meetings, of any size, are so critical.

Being an AA loner and a gay person meant a secondary level of isolation.[5] Feeling alone, feeling different—these things can be more real for a loner. There was a very palpable sense of, *yes, I am the only one.*

I would change the pronouns [substituting "she" for "he"] when I shared at a meeting and that made it difficult for me to feel I was being rigorously honest. But when I took the Third Step and started to develop a relationship with a Higher Power, I felt my Higher Power understood why I had to change the pronouns. My Higher Power allowed me, and forgave me if that was necessary, and understood that my sobriety was more important than making political statements in meetings.

I found that my loneliness could help others. At about fifteen years of sobriety, I had to declare bankruptcy at the same time I ended a six-year relationship, went through an IRS audit, and lost my home. Through those experiences, I've been able to share with others who have gone through bankruptcy, or lost their home, or their relationship.

In 1980, at Living Sober, someone asked me to lead a workshop, and I said that I would. The workshop turned out to be "Sex and Sobriety for Men." So many people showed up for that workshop that they had to move it to the auditorium! There I was, a man from Pink

Hill, North Carolina, talking to 300 men in San Francisco about sex and sobriety. I discovered I had something worthwhile to share—that my experience, my sobriety, and my relationship with my Higher Power could be useful for somebody else.

At about that time I started writing to other gay loners. Those letters were a kind of an ongoing journal, as well as AA Fourth and Fifth Steps. It was a cleansing process that helped me become more aware of who I was. Sometimes the people I corresponded with would ask, "Why write to me? Why send *me* handwritten letters?" and then I'd pass on what Tom told me the first time he sent me that registration form with his handwritten note.

"Doug, if we put on Living Sober this year, if we have all those meetings, and make all those thousands of cups of coffee, and the only thing that happens is that you stay sober, then this whole Roundup will have been worth it." That's the message: "You are worth it," I tell them. "If I write pages of letters, and nothing else happens but that you stay sober, then every page of every letter is worth it because you are worth it."

I might also tell them something else I heard early in sobriety: If you want somebody to do something for you, do that thing for somebody else. If you're lonely, help take away someone else's loneliness. If you want attention, if you need fellowship, reach out, someway, somehow. You may not know what good your letter, phone call, or e-mail may do, but [your] Higher Power knows.

Sometimes I'd see someone I corresponded with at an AA conference. . . . Whenever I saw these people, it was a joyous homecoming. We'd talk about our lives, about the things we'd said in our letters. We were family, getting together again! It was fellowship, a long-distance bond in time and geography that, many times, lasted for years. Until, now that Tom has passed away, as far as I know, everybody I used to write letters to has died. Every one of them. [We sit quietly awhile.]

Whatever is going on, whatever you have to do to get through it—every Fifth Step you have to do, every Ninth Step amend you have to make, every time you pray—all the things you do for yourself in recovery are worth doing. Because you are worth it, you are worth doing this for. . . .

Geri C.

[Geri got sober in Portland, Oregon, in 1978.]

When I was eighteen I went into the army. I kissed a girl for the first time at Fort McClellan, Alabama, and I was so freaked out that I went to the post library and looked up homosexuality. The catalog said, "see Witchcraft; Demonology." [I thought,] *Oh my god!* . . .

My experience being a lesbian in the military was so horrendous— let alone any of the other things that were happening from 1967 to 1970. It was such a turbulent time in my life, and in the world. I marched in my first civil rights march in May 1968. I was in Alabama when Martin Luther King was killed. I was on my way to [Washington DC,] when Robert Kennedy was shot. I was there the weekend they brought his body back to Washington.[6]

When we first get to AA, most of us aren't exactly brimming with open-mindedness and willingness. . . . I confused spirituality and religion for a long time because the revolutionary path I was on did not include fundamentalist religious doctrine, which is what I thought AA's Twelve Steps were. I'd hear people in meetings say, "I'm grateful to be an alcoholic," or, "I asked God for a parking place, and I found one!" I'd think, *You need an introduction to dialectical materialism.* I love that line by Herbert Spencer in the AA Big Book, about contempt prior to investigation.[7] . . . I am so grateful to the atheists and agnostics in AA who paved a path for me.

I was a social service worker when I went into treatment. As a community activist, I had been trying to build support for women. I was working on the Women's Mental Health Project. . . . The woman I worked with was my best drinking buddy. We drank beer all day and wrote grants together.

I knew of two treatment centers for alcoholism in Portland at the time: the Care Unit at Physicians and Surgeons Hospital, where I went, and Raleigh Hills. Raleigh Hills used aversion therapy.[8] I used to drink beer and watch Gail Storms talk about throwing up [Storms was a former-patient-turned-spokesperson for Raleigh Hills] and think, *What a bad idea. If throwing up got you sober, I'd be sober already!* I was a sick, hungover, and kind of drunk addict, with complications of many different kinds of chemicals.

I had a lot of fears about going into treatment. I had two uncles in state hospitals for the insane on the back alcoholic wards. That's what I knew about addiction. I'd been a medic in the army, but alcoholism was not addressed there. Everyone drank. I was taking care of blown-up bodies from Vietnam. I did not know how to deal with what was going on. Normal drinking was never anything I aspired to.

At the Care Unit, I told them that if I was going to stay there, they could not lock me up, and that they could not tell me I drank and used because I was queer. . . . I was told that that wouldn't be an issue, and my treatment counselor referred me to the two gay AA meetings in Portland at the time, held at the Metropolitan Community Church. I had a hard time at those meetings, mostly because of my politics.

One time, it was International Women's Day, and I was all hot to trot, and I went up to the secretary. "Happy International Women's Day!" I said.

She looked at me. "Oh? Is it?"

And I thought, *Jesus Christ. How am I supposed to take over the world with these people?* They seemed to be totally into this God business, this "Him" thing. This Alcoholics Anonymous stuff sounded like poppycock. "Turn It Over." "Easy Does It." Where do they get this *mishegoss* [foolishness]? Hallmark cards?

I'm a balker. I'm the one that goes, "Whaaa!" but does it anyway. *[Laughing]* I'm willing—I'm just a *screaming* willing person. . . .

In 1980, a friend took me to a lesbian AA meeting in Portland. It was held at your house. I remember sitting on the floor, reading aloud from a weird book about "Step Three." It was written by a man, whose whole point seemed to be that we should believe in God. I thought you were the weirdest lesbian I'd ever seen.

Oh, it was very confusing because we are reading literature written in 1935 that is sexist, and classist, yet universal. I had so much translation to do, to try and sort out who I was. And it didn't work anymore for me to switch "God" to "Goddess." I wasn't down with that kind of veggie, femme stuff, either. I was a Marxist, for god's sake!

I banged around for a year. I kept getting loaded, and I kept coming back. . . . I was in a rage. . . . One day there was another guy having a fit in a meeting, and we left together. He had a crowbar in his car, and we took turns using it to beat the "Easy Does It" sticker off his bumper.

When I first got clean I had such guilt and shame for the people I'd hurt. It wasn't the rippin' and the runnin'. It was that I'd been loved by wonderful people, and I had no idea what was going on in my own life. In the 1970s, some lesbians from the Socialist Health Workers Group I was in tried to confront me about my using.

"Just don't use so *much,* Geri. We love you," they said, but they didn't know how to help me. Two of them were nurses, and I love nurses. My deal with nurses was to find a woman who would take care of me, while I took care of the world—find two or three of them because I was too much for one person. So, I had all this guilt and shame. . . .

As lesbians and gay men, we didn't have models. I slept with women, so I thought I must know how to get along with them. We had no boundaries. I came from the generation whose motto was "sex, drugs, and rock 'n' roll." Who knew the B word? I learned about that in recovery. I didn't understand that just because I had emotional and sexual relationships with women didn't mean I knew about intimacy, or healthy relationships.

When I got sober, I had a strong gay and lesbian community I was connected to, but I could not go to them for support. Bars, drugs, and alcohol were a big part of our community. They still are. So where do you go to have a good time? Everybody I knew and loved was still drinking and using. It was a huge loss. Even the people who didn't have a problem with alcohol or drugs were surrounded by it. There was an incredible tolerance for drunk and loaded behavior in the gay community.

In Narcotics Anonymous, I've never felt the need for a gay meeting because the preamble includes the words "regardless of sexual identity." It says it right there. I also find fewer class distinctions in NA than in [AA]. It's just the nature of the beast. You know how addicts are viewed by some people in this culture, even though alcohol is one water molecule away from ether. If they used the same criteria in the Federal Drug Schedule to judge alcohol as they do other drugs, it would take two keys to get to it in a narcotics locker. It's such a powerful chemical.

A lot of people think NA's First Step says, "We admitted we were powerless over drugs." But it doesn't. It begins, "We admitted we were powerless over addiction." Because our disease is addiction.

Narcotics Anonymous has built a worldwide fellowship based on the concept of total abstinence—which takes care of whatever else you might get your happy little derriere into in recovery.

There have been those pioneers in AA and NA who understood at a deeper level that in the beginning we need to find people who are like us. There has to be a place for us to come together. It's not that people are exclusionary. I see it as the difference between uniformity and unanimity, and we don't all have to be the same. We're not all the same! But I have never wanted to go just to gay meetings or just to women's meetings. I was taught a lot by people I wouldn't have gotten loaded with. I received patience and tolerance from people who, from the outside, didn't seem anything like me. I learned to cry from watching men. I [too] was broken in that way.

There are people who think I'm sick, who think I'm sinful, who think by the very nature of who I love that I am less-than. Do those people exist in twelve-step rooms? Of course. We're all raised with this. We have to unlearn it. I remember being at a young people's conference once where a speaker told gay jokes from the podium, and I was devastated. I thought, *If I don't belong here where can I go?*

One day my friend Mari and I went to a meeting at the Portland Alano Club. Mari was great. We got clean together, and she modeled stuff for me. We sat there and listened while the speaker told racist jokes. Mari leaned over and said, "What's the matter, Geri? You're white, aren't you? What have *you* got to bitch about? I'm a lesbian and I'm black. Oh my *god!*" . . .

And there's been that whole phenomenon in the lesbian community about people [who] used to be lesbians. What do you do if you were always a lesbian, and all of a sudden you fall in love with a man? So what? What are we afraid of? People in recovery sometimes examine their sexuality. Recovery is like taking yourself apart bone by bone. You have to know who you are.

My little utopian dream is that people can just exist and be who they are. But we don't live in a world like that, so we have these little boxes, where we're women or we're black or we're addicts or we're Latinos. We speak different languages. Our economic class is different. But the fabulous thing about the Twelve Step Traditions is that none of that matters.

When I go to AA meetings now, I identify myself as an alcoholic. I used to talk about drugs like crazy, and be as outrageous as I could. That was part of my defense. Lesbians and gay men are some of the most emotionally well-defended people in the world. We have powerful defense mechanisms because we need them to survive. . . . I needed that kind of survival technique to exist in a world that tells me I'm not okay. A defense mechanism is there to protect you.

. . . Our defense mechanisms protect us, but we can hurt people with them as well. When we view ourselves as victims, we can do to others what has been done to us. We become reactionary. For example, I used to call men "boys" because I'd been called "girl." So I have to look at that stuff in me. What part do I have in it? . . .

Geri, how did you get from that emotional place where you took a crowbar to an "Easy Does It" bumper sticker, to where you are today?

I think what happened, despite my ranting and raving, was that nobody turned me out. Here I was, this totally sensitive, weenie-thing, screaming her brains out because I couldn't cry. Gradually, my heart softened, and one day I noticed that people had been loving and tolerating *me*, that I was the one people wouldn't ordinarily mix with. And look how wonderful they'd been! I realized then that what I wanted was what had already been given to me. And that I should give that away.

I once heard a man speak who said, "You have to know yourself, so you can be yourself, so you can get over yourself." I was always trying to get over myself and I didn't even know who I was. I have continued to write inventories to find out more [about] who I am. Some of the deepest inventories I've written have been about my best not being good enough. Oh, I have my street persona, yet underneath is this vulnerable woman, who wants to live with her heart open. Today, I choose to live with my heart open. . . .

Judy S.

[Judy lives in Wilmington, Illinois, a small community about thirty miles south of Joliet, Illinois. She came out as a lesbian in 1993.]

The last couple of years I drank I knew something was seriously wrong with me. I thought I had some kind of mental illness, but not alcoholism. I entered treatment in 1978. I went to my first meeting to make them happy, but it only took a couple of meetings before I was pretty sure there was an answer there for me.

In 1992, I met Nancy. We worked on a women's AA conference together, and one day, after we'd been friends for about a year, she came out to me. *[Laughing]* I was very surprised . . . but I wasn't in horror because I'd spent the last eight years of my married life trying to talk myself out of being a lesbian.

Nancy introduced me to Karen, who was straight and had been sober a long time, and she'd sponsored many lesbians in AA. I came out to her, and she became my sponsor. She was a rock. I was nearing the end of my marriage, and I was coming to grips with my sexual orientation, and feeling half nuts.

I finally decided, *Yes, I am a lesbian. And yes, I am going to get divorced.* I'd never been with a woman sexually; the only other gay person I knew was Nancy. The only thing I knew about the lesbian and gay community were the pictures of the [Gay] Pride Parade they showed on the Chicago news for thirty seconds every year.

Karen said I could be married and still be a lesbian. It made sense to her, but it made no sense to me. And we disagreed to the point where she didn't want to sponsor me anymore, so our relationship ended. It was a big loss.

Things were moving very quickly. I moved from my home that I shared with my husband and took my two daughters and rented an apartment. My perspective was changing—roles, labels—everything seemed to be taking a different slant to it. I've always gone to meetings on a regular basis, but this was a period I didn't go because I got it in my head somehow that AA was going to take this slant too. For weeks I told myself that I had better gear up, because, like everything else, AA was going to change, and I should just go to a meeting and learn how to deal with it. I finally went to one, one where I knew people. And sitting there, the words of my first sponsor came to me.

"Judy," she said, "I'm going to tell you something about AA. You either deal yourself in, or you deal yourself out." And that truth went deeper that day than it ever had before. I realized the shift hadn't happened with AA, that my role and my identity as an AA member would not change. I was so grateful that it was up to *me* to continue to be in AA, [that] it was up to *me* to say, "Yes, I'm in, and you can't kick me out."

In 1995, I started going to the Friday night women's meeting at the gay Alano Club in Forest Park. People were serious about staying sober, and there was a solid core of about fifteen women, with a wide range of sobriety and backgrounds, but the third year [that I attended that meeting], over a period of about two months, different women started coming in, and, suddenly, people were just coupling up! After that, the group got very small. I stopped attending, and it fell apart within a couple of years.

Had you begun to get a sense of a gay community outside of AA before that happened?

A little bit. I'd met my partner, Jill, at a party, and we had some social contact through friends of hers. There was a bar in Franklin Park, called Temptations where we'd go with the Friday Night Women's Group and dance. No one slipped at that bar, and we had a good time. But then they changed the music, and we got older, and we just didn't know how to dance to that music, so we quit going.

Maybe once every two months, I'd go to a straight meeting just to see how it was. I felt like I had a place there, but I didn't feel like I could be real free. I wouldn't sit there and say, "Oh, my partner, Jill," or anything about her, and I didn't want to say "my friend."

In 2001, Jill and I moved to Wilmington, and that's when I connected more with other women in AA. Now I'm working on the [Midwest] Woman-to-Woman [AA] conference. Wilmington's a little podunk town where it's mostly good-old-boy, and I'm not exaggerating. It would be nice to have some friends here in town, where you don't have to drive an hour. Before we moved, we used to love driving down to Chicago. Eight hours driving time and then we'd be there for four or five hours.

The gay and lesbian AA community in Joliet, about twenty-five minutes from here, is very small. At the Monday night [gay AA] meeting there are maybe five or six [people], but there's not a solid core. At one point, the men decided they wanted to have their own meeting. Then they realized they missed the women, so they invited us to their meeting to make it a little more interesting.

I haven't come out at [regular AA] meetings in Joliet because the parking lot I have to walk through [to get to] many of these meetings—I don't want to be a statistic of a hate crime. That's not homophobic on my part. That's the reality. In Joliet, particularly at the Alano Club, probably at one out of five meetings you're going to hear a homophobic remark—very blatant and very clear.

The first meeting specifically for lesbians I ever went to was at a women's conference in Milwaukee. There was just one lesbian meeting, and someone kept taking the sign [announcing it] down, and someone [else] kept putting it back up. Out of about 250 women [at the conference], there were eight of us there. Everyone said how long they'd been sober, and when they came out, and I just sat there. Everyone else had come out in their first few months of sobriety. I was sober fifteen years before I came out! I never thought I'd be embarrassed to say how long I'd been sober.

I'm on the program committee for this year's Woman-to-Woman conference, and about half the women wanted meetings for lesbians and half didn't. I was one who didn't want to have to have special meetings. I want to be mainstream. It wasn't that I wanted to go into the closet. It was, "Let's be together. We are all a part of this conference, so let's be in it!" But someone else's viewpoint was that new people, or someone like me, who was sober longer just coming out, would not feel comfortable speaking freely, which is true. And that's why lesbian meetings got voted in.

When . . . the steering committee [heard our decision], they bucked. Oh, did they buck! Well, I shouldn't say they; it was just one person who didn't want any meeting identified as lesbian, who didn't even want the word mentioned. It took about three meetings to hammer it out, but she was voted down almost unanimously. So there are going to be lesbian meetings at the conference, one each day. . . .

Have you noticed a difference in being thought of as an "old-timer" in the gay AA community, compared to the larger AA community?

In the gay AA community, I'm put on a pedestal. The Monday night crew had a rainbow banquet, and they made a special point of getting a twenty-three-year coin and giving it to me. They were getting a big kick out of it and it really touched me, but—It's that not-fitting-in thing. . . . My friend Eileen even said to me, "Judy, there's a kind of aura about you." I told her, "Eileen, come live with me for a week. Believe me. The aura won't be there!" I want them to see the real me.

When I was first sober, I wanted so badly to be normal that I chose the path defined by society: to get married, to have children. Today I rely more on what I think is going to add to my life. I worry less about what people are thinking. I'm more settled with myself, the roles that I have—as an AA member, as a lesbian, as a mother—have become more integrated.

I look forward to the day I can speak at an open AA meeting and tell my story and be comfortable. I've been asked to speak, but I've backed off because coming out is a big part of my AA story, and I don't know how to tell my story without telling that part. It would sound stilted, too careful. But that day will come, *[laughing]* although I might be eighty. No, I hope not!

Lee V.

[Lee got sober in Houston, Texas.]

The night of Christmas 1977, I had my last drink. I ended up in a hospital with palpitations and arrhythmia, and I thought I was having a heart attack. It never occurred to me that I might have a drinking problem. It still overwhelms me, because sobriety was not in my plans. A guy I used to drink with took me to my first meeting. We went to Lambda Houston [Houston's gay Alano Club]. It was their first or second meeting, in their own little clubhouse.

I didn't know anything about AA, and this first group was like a secret society. Everyone was terrified that people were going to come kick in the doors and go after them, they were going to come shoot the queers, because that had been going on for so long in Houston. So it was very exciting to be in AA!

I was very shaky. "We're so glad you're here," they told me. "Keep coming back," and I thought, *These people have a group, and they want me in it? That's crazy.*

The first Lambda group started out in a little two-bedroom house. We told each other where we were by word-of-mouth. Nobody had any time [in AA] when I came in. Jerry D. had nine years, and he was the phenomenon. Jerry told us it was okay to be ourselves, that we weren't bad for [starting a gay AA group], and we believed him.

Coming from New York, Houston was a major shock. I'd been part of the first gathering that came together [in New York] after Stonewall, and the first Christopher Street Pride Parade. So here I land in Houston, and Houston is a cow town. I kid you not, people would ride to 7-Eleven on a *horse.* The late 1970s was a dangerous time [to be gay] in Houston. Gay people were getting shot at in the street. . . . There were these garden-type gay bars, and they would shoot at people through the fences. I knew a man who was hit by a flying bullet. Walking down the street you could get caught in the crossfire.

It was still such a backward place, and I was so open, and so out. I was from New York, and I knew everything! I was just all smart, you know. I'd walk into the Lambda clubhouse and try to talk to these people, and they were so kind. They'd say to me, "Girl, you talk funny!" And I'd say, "No, you talk funny!" And we'd have this little ongoing thing. They saved my life, these people. I feel blessed to have found that group in Houston, or that it found me, however it happened. I'd thought, *Aw, they're just a bunch of wusses,* but, instead, they were my heroes.

Lambda Houston became an enormous group. We bought a garage that had been a mechanics shop. [To raise money,] we put on yard sales, bake sales, and we had drag shows where we'd sell the clothes off the drag queens' backs. We were having a grand time! Decorating the place was a riot. Four or five guys were interior decorators, and they'd walk in and say, "I'm never coming back here. I can't stay sober in *this* color!" We laughed, and we painted, and we got involved.

I remember being shocked at how huge Lambda Houston had become. People would come in, and say, "Wow! You guys have something we've never seen before, not a place to drink, but a place to *go.*" And it became the place to go in Houston. Gay people would say, "Haven't you been to Lambda?"

I started going to lots of meetings, and I got a sponsor. I didn't want a gay sponsor. I didn't trust that they wouldn't end up being a Thirteenth Step call [that the relationship would become sexual] on me, or them. I told this woman I was gay, and she said, "I don't care," and I said, "Good," and we became sponsor/sponsee.

"Where do you go to meetings?" she asked me.

"I go to Lambda."

"I've heard about that place."

"Why don't you come Saturday night? We have a big speaker meet—"

"I'd love to!" she said, and pretty soon, other straight people started coming. Then we started inviting straight people to speak, so it started integrating nicely and people came together.

But the minute you headed out of central Houston, into the countryside, oh, it got really ugly. There were all kinds of comments about "the queers coming here." One night my sponsor and I went to a meeting, and as we walked in I heard a woman say, "And here she is, followed by that little queer she hangs out with." One night this guy came up to me. His name was Bubba.

Bubba said, "Honey, are you having trouble with your lady?"

"As a matter of fact, I am." I said. I was dumbfounded.

"Darlin', I've been there. I know how sad that is."

"My God, Bubba," I said. "You scared the hell out of me!"

He was the most darling man. So this was the other side of AA—where you had some real sweet Bubbas.

Lambda Houston was the first group to put our heads out and say that we wanted to have a hospitality suite for gay people at the 1980 International AA Convention in New Orleans, and they said yes! I worked there pouring coffee, the usual, and we were thrilled to be there—New Orleans, the Superdome. Here we were, doing this AA thing, and the world had come to our doorstep just to be a part of it. One night they announced, "We have a gay hospitality suite here, for those of you who'd like to stop by," from the main stage, and that brought tears to our eyes because nobody ever dreamed this would be accepted.

The hospitality suite was always packed. People would wander in and say, "Well, what have we got here?"

"We're the Lambda Group of Houston," we'd tell them.

"Great!" they'd say, but half of them didn't know what that meant. Some people said, "You go right ahead and be gay. It's okay with me," and we'd say, "Okay. We'll do that."

One man came in and said, "I don't know who you people are, or where you came from. I've been in AA for thirty-eight years—" He started to cry. "I've been gay all my life, and I've never told the truth and—I'm so scared. But you people have given me the courage to say who I am." I still choke up when I think about him.

I grew up in New York City, and the Village was always right there. I've been out since I was a kid. I mean, I've never been in. I started going to the Village when I was seventeen. It was scary for me because the lesbians [who] were visible in the Village were not exactly what I wanted to be. They wore men's clothing. They strapped down their chests with banding and wore men's underwear. That's what I came into, and I didn't know there was any other way. It was only later that I realized I could be my own person and didn't have to emulate anybody. But that took a bit of doing.

The first lesbian bar I stepped foot into was the Bagatelle. It was quite a nice place, and they had a bouncer to protect the women coming and going. Other bars had bouncers, but nothing compared to Eddie. He was huge! Eddie's job was to protect the clients from people coming in and getting ugly, which was not unusual in New York City. So, if you were not a lesbian, or with a lesbian, you'd probably never get in. [The bouncers] were there for our protection—protection for queers—and they got paid quite a bit. Up until the early 1990s, most of the bars in New York City were Mafia-owned. The Bagatelle was probably Mafia-owned. I can only say probably because, at the time, I didn't have a lot of political snap.

There was a Bar Guild, where the owners of all the bars came together and tossed out ideas on how to keep the bars open. So we always had good interaction. In 1973 we decided we were going to have a Gay Pride kind of thing, but we didn't know what it should look like. I was working as a bartender in the Village and my boss decided to be part of this.

Everybody was kind of fighting; there was a lot of in-fighting going on, with people saying things like, "You're doing it wrong," and, "You're the wrong kind of queer"—you're the wrong kind of this and the wrong kind of that. I remember thinking how funny we were—that we were really all in the same boat, trying to sink it together.

My friend Nancy and I got very involved, going around and hustling the other bars to get involved, and we finally pulled it off. Then they asked us to be parade marshals. We didn't know what that meant, so we said, "Sure!" Nancy and I would volunteer for anything. They trained us in marshaling the crowd, nonviolent marshaling, like moving people back with linking arms.

Then on the day of the parade, the marshal came down and said, "We would like you and Nancy to be on-stage bodyguards for the entertainment." "Grand!" we say. "We're going to be bodyguards!" And off we go. And when we get to Central Park, we are escorted on stage as bodyguards for two unknown talents: a piano player named Barry Manilow and a singer named Bette Midler. Bette had just started singing at the tubs,[9] and we were totally taken with her.

I used to open a bar at noon in the Village, and after that I'd run into Bette on my way to work. One day, this guy who was walking with me said, "Look. Over there. It's Bette Midler!"

Bette sees me and says, "Lee! How are you?"

"Oh my god," he says. "She knows you?"

"Well," I say, "only because I was her personal bodyguard."

[Laughing] So that's part of coming out. I was always very out there. I was never too fearful of what was going to happen to me. Crazy, a little bit. When I got sober, I came back to the Village. I ran into lots of people I drank with, and we were night and day apart. "God," they said, "you've really changed." I never went into the details of it, but I had changed.

Now I live in San Miguel de Allende, Mexico. There are a lot of people here with long-term sobriety—people who still have sponsors, people who still go to meetings, who still ask for help and reach out to other people. I was taught that when someone walks through the doors of AA, you go up and introduce yourself and welcome them. So we do a lot of that here in San Miguel, and we have an enormous number of newcomers.

I'm very willing to take the hand of the newcomer. For a while, I didn't feel I had a connection, but I've found that the longer I'm in AA, the more connection I have with everybody. I'm willing to take the call that comes in the middle of the night. Some people say, "Don't call me if you've been drinking." But I say, "Call me." Because I remember hearing things when I was drunk. That's how I keep my program going.

Today I'm not hiding out behind anything. I feel comfortable growing older, getting a little bit older your behavior is better. I was at a meeting in Florida one time, and this guy was reading the newspaper. Right in the middle of the meeting he announces, "Goddamn queer! They should have killed him instead of just beating him up!" People were horrified.

I went up to him after [the meeting]. "You know, you and I talk a lot in AA, and I'm gay."

"I didn't know that."

"Well, you even like some of us," I said. "Maybe you want to rethink your thinking."

When I was newly sober, a man asked me after a meeting if I'd come work at the New York Psychiatric Hospital. We went out to coffee after the meeting.

"How long you been sober?"

"Less than a year," I said.

"Oh, no. No. You can't do it. I thought you had more time." Then he says, "How about volunteering?"

"Okay. What do you want me to do?"

I started bringing a meeting into the hospital and driving these guys to meetings outside. We had this huge van [that could hold] between twelve and fifteen. These guys were from Harlem, from the streets. They were really something else, these guys. I thought they were wonderful. We bonded, me and most of them.

One afternoon, the director of the unit says, "Lee, I'd like you to do something really different. Could you, and maybe two or three other people, come talk about gay AA?"

So that night [I] and my sponsor, and a couple of other people, put on a panel discussion meeting at the hospital. We talked about special interest groups, and how some people weren't straight, but in order to act straight they had to get drunk. We put on this whole thing.

And I was terrified because here are these guys I knew, these street guys, who were really scary, sitting there with their mouths hanging open. They started asking a lot of questions, and pretty soon everybody was talking.

After the meeting, this Puerto Rican guy comes up to me. He goes, "What happened? You stopped being my friend."

"Um, no. Why?"

"Why couldn't you tell me your truth? You think I don't love you? 'Cause you're a dyke? You think I don't love you 'cause you're a bull dagger?"

I started to cry.

"We love you," he says. "We don't care who you are. We love you."

And here I was, thinking I was doing some big, hotshot deal, [bringing a meeting into the hospital], and I got all the benefits.

Chapter 15

On Our Way:
A Conversation with Lillene Fifield

Introduction

Lillene Fifield's 1975 study, *On My Way to Nowhere: Alienated, Isolated, and Drunk, an Analysis of Alcoholism in the Gay and Lesbian Community,* is a landmark work in the alcoholism field. In 1974, Fifield led the effort to found the Alcoholism Center for Women (ACW) in Los Angeles. She has served on the California Women's Commission on Alcoholism, the State of California Alcoholism Advisory Board, and the NALGAP Advisory Board. At the California Alcoholism Foundation, she worked to measure and address homophobia and sexism in treatment facilities. Today she is a lecturer and consultant, and maintains a private psychotherapy practice in Southern California.

Lillene Fifield

When I was twenty-one I moved to Los Angeles. I found friends, and a peer group. In the 1950s and 1960s, a gay person's social life was centered mostly in bars. There was nowhere else to go. I moved back to Kansas City in 1966, and when I returned to Los Angeles in 1969, I was amazed to discover that some of my old friends had drinking problems.

I began looking for ways to meet people other than in a bar. I heard rumblings about a place on Melrose Avenue called the Gay Libera-

The History of Gay People in Alcoholics Anonymous
Published by The Haworth Press, Inc., 2007. All rights reserved.
doi:10.1300/5699_15

tion Front, and I visited there, but found only men. It was hard to relate to them because I was looking to make women friends. Although I was Jewish, I discovered the Metropolitan Community Church, which at that time was being held in Troy Perry's house. Then, in 1971, I found my way to the Gay Community Services Center of Los Angeles. It had just opened, in a funky old Victorian house on Wilshire Boulevard. It was beautiful! It felt like home. My involvement at the center changed my life.

I wanted to be a community organizer. And I realized that if the center was to survive as an organization, we could not do it on donations alone. I wanted to learn about grant writing, and program design and development, and evaluation. I spent my second year of graduate school in a fieldwork placement learning exactly those things.

The University of Southern California (USC) Regional Research Institute is important because, later, when we wrote the grant for the Alcoholism Program for Women, the institute signed on as the program's primary investigator. We were given a little over a million dollars for three years. And in 1974, that was a great deal of money. It was the largest grant ever made to a new program, to a women's program, and to a lesbian program. USC's involvement was significant in it being granted.

A year or so earlier, Don Kilhefner and Morris Kight, the founders of the Gay Community Center, had founded the Van Ness House for recovering gay alcoholics. The three of us started writing grants for the center's many volunteer-run programs. The programs that exist at the Gay and Lesbian Community Services Center today have their roots back in those early grants. One of the greater needs in the gay and lesbian community was the high incidence of alcoholism. The center had an opportunity when we heard from Rita Saenz—Rita was then an NIAAA consultant[1]—that money was available to start a women's program. Rita is currently director of the California Department of Social Services.

Brenda Weathers and I, along with a group of support people that included a woman named Travis Foote, worked very carefully on the NIAAA grant, and it was finally funded in 1974. While we were celebrating, we suddenly realized that I'd forgotten to ask for money to buy beds, sheets, towels, and dishes! *[Laughing]* Fortunately, we were able to get a little additional money for those things.

So that's how the Alcoholism Center for Women (ACW) came into being. ACW remains today in its original location on South Alvarado [Street] in Los Angeles, where it has served women, primarily lesbian women and women of color, continuously since 1974. It is a landmark for our community. We are a young community, and it is a significant part of our history.

In those days, Alcoholics Anonymous was not the friendliest place for a gay or lesbian person. Homophobia forced many gay people to lie about their most basic identity—in an atmosphere where recovery is dependent on brutal honesty—so there existed a huge contradiction.

In 1975, money became available from the Los Angeles County Office of Alcohol Programs to do a study on alcoholism in the gay and lesbian community. That grant, made to the Gay and Lesbian Center, enabled me to do the first research on the incidence and characteristics of alcoholism in our community and the recovery options available to gay and lesbian alcoholics.

The original report, titled *On My Way to Nowhere: Alienated, Isolated, and Drunk, an Analysis of Alcoholism in the Gay and Lesbian Community*, was the definitive work at the time. It later became known as the Fifield Report, and a few of the original 100 copies of the 250-page report can still be found in libraries and archives. In 1977, David Latham and I wrote a condensed version for the State of California Office of Publications. They promised a publication run of 20,000, but I saw only about 500 copies.

Two aspects of that report were very significant. We interviewed program directors and staff from approximately fifty alcohol recovery programs in Los Angeles County, and we administered an instrument[2] to determine the degree of homophobia in those organizations. [This was] the first time this had ever been done. It included scales that measured rigidity because we wanted to look at whether fixed or rigid attitudes about other things would affect a person's attitudes about gays and lesbians. And we included an instrument to measure sexism because, we hypothesized, if a person was rigid and sexist, they were also likely to be homophobic, and, of course, our hypothesis proved itself, overwhelmingly.

When we got the results from the interviews with agency directors and staff, and found the high degree of rigidity, sexist attitudes, and homophobia, it reinforced what recovering people were saying about their attempts to recover in non–gay and lesbian programs.

Another significant part of the study involved asking gay and lesbian people about their experiences in AA, and Alcoholics Together. Alcoholics Together had obtained space in an area of Los Angeles called Silver Lake, and immediately meetings were going practically around the clock. For the first time, there were places to refer recovering gay and lesbian people [to], where they did not have to worry about encountering homophobia.

Many reported [on our survey] that they'd tried to maintain sobriety in AA and found it too difficult to have to maintain a dual identity there. Again, the statistics were overwhelming, in terms of the homophobia the interviewees reported experiencing in AA. And they reinforced our findings because they repeatedly reported that they'd attempted to recover in non–gay or lesbian settings and failed. Those who subsequently attained sobriety in gay-identified treatment programs, and attended AT meetings, reported finally getting and staying sober.

Some people say AA was slow to change, but I don't think so. I think AA made some major changes during that five-year period. Attitudes changed greatly toward gay and lesbian recovering people. Attitudes toward women and [their] traditional roles also changed. And as newcomers came in, they picked up a different perspective, and it carried itself forth.

Information from the Fifield Report was slow in getting published. Some of it was carried in small articles in local papers, and quotes found their way into many texts and journal articles. Getting information disseminated in the gay and lesbian community was more difficult. In fact, when the study on alcoholism in the gay community first came out, it was trashed.

The *Journal of Homosexuality* rejected printing the initial articles, which I thought was very interesting. In the letter of rejection I received, the methodology we used was challenged. My undergraduate degree is in sociology and social welfare and I brought that and my social work background into my research. Social survey research methodology, which is a perfectly legitimate form, is very different from traditional psychology methodology, which uses control groups.

But the underlying reason behind the rejection, as we were told in discussions that occurred, had to do with the alarming statistics in the report. Many folks did not want to see information published that said one-third of the community drank to problem-drinking proportions, and 24 percent were, by definition, alcoholics. In the mid-1970s, when people were trying to present a more positive image of gay identity, most community leadership felt our good reputation and image was assaulted enough.

The original Fifield Study was replicated by the Menninger Foundation in 1981 in four communities in Kansas and Missouri, and they came up with exactly the same statistics—exactly the same. It was replicated again in San Francisco in the mid-1980s—not the whole study, which was a huge undertaking, but parts of it—and in San Francisco they found that the statistics were still the same, but that the drug of choice was starting to shift. Polydrug use is more prevalent in our community now, and [that] would be the most significant change I would point to between the 1970s and today.

Between 1974 and 1978, we had [an] impact on a lot of different fronts. I served on the Los Angeles County Alcoholism Advisory Board where a lot of grants were made to treatment programs in Los Angeles County. I was also president of the California Alcoholism Foundation and served on their board. The foundation provided trainings in the 1970s and 1980s to alcohol treatment programs throughout California. I was also part of the founding of the California Women's Commission on Alcoholism and one of their first cochairs, and the commission made a major commitment to dealing with sexism and homophobia. Through the work of these two fine groups, we were able to include a lot of information on sexism and homophobia as our membership interacted with many different agencies around the state.

Information was reaching treatment programs, which meant that people coming into treatment were exposed to a much broader perspective, [one] that included information about lesbian and gay alcoholics. As those people left recovery programs and moved into AA, they brought a different set of attitudes with them. Much of the staff in treatment agencies are themselves folks in recovery, and many of the treatment programs utilized AA foundations in their design.

Wow. I am beginning to see just how broad, and deliberate, your strategy was.

To create lasting change, attitudes have to change. You have to change what people do, and what they think. You don't do research for research's sake! You must have a focus, a purpose, and an intention for that research. It is not enough to have a hypothesis! If the hypothesis is proved true, what then, can we do about it?

When people get together to make change, there is a model with which to do that. It's not just that you wave placards and scream and yell. You need to come up with clear ideas about what people can do to help themselves achieve what they ultimately want to achieve. Then it's very easy for people to go the direction one needs to go in order for change to happen.

George M____ told me that he'd saved a series of articles by Randy Shilts on alcoholism in the gay community, published by The Advocate *in the 1970s. Years later, while planning the National Council on Alcoholism's annual conference, he discovered that they were based on the work of someone named Lillene Fifield. George told me he tracked you down in Oregon and invited you to speak.*

Following the *Journal of Homosexuality*'s refusal to print the article, it was very difficult to get the word out, and very disheartening to have that kind of rejection. Randy Shilts, who has since passed on, was known to be a very courageous author and writer. He would tackle subjects that weren't popular because they needed to be written about. Randy came to me and said he'd gotten a copy of the study and was concerned that it had gotten very little publication space. He wanted to do a series of articles on alcoholism and asked if I was agreeable. I absolutely jumped with joy at the idea!

Randy did extensive interviews with me and wrote what I think is the finest piece of investigative journalism of his career. As you know, he later went on to do the same thing with AIDS.[3] He spent a good part of his career doing that very courageous and very legitimate work of uncovering things that other people would rather not have uncovered. He wrote the articles, and because of *The Advocate's* wide circulation, the information finally reached the audiences we wanted it to reach, which of course were gay and lesbian people, as well as other folk.

By 1979, I had been on the front lines for almost ten years. My whole life had been about community organizing, and building, and moving and shaking, and I was burned out. I decided to move to Oregon and retire and grow my own food, you know, that whole thing, and that is where George found me.

It was very exciting to hear that there was to be a track on alcoholism in the gay and lesbian community at the conference. I went to Seattle with my co-author David Latham, who helped me write the condensed version. He picked me up in Roseburg and the two of us rode up to Seattle on his motorcycle, a trip of about 500 miles. We stayed at the Seattle YMCA. David has also since died of AIDS.

It was in Seattle that your message was finally received at a national level.

I received a huge applause—that was very heartwarming—and gratitude—that was so rewarding.

I don't know whether George told you this. But after the speech, so many people came forward with incredible stories about what they were doing as a result of the work, that I just stood up there, kind of bawling. People told me how they'd gotten mimeographs or [photo-] copies of the study and used them to lobby for treatment program funding in their states, how they'd used the results to support their attempts to change attitudes at non–gay and lesbian service providers and treatment agencies. I just sat on the steps to the podium, listening and appreciating the impact the work was having. I was overwhelmed, and deeply touched that the truth had gotten out. This was validation of a major information shift within the recovery community, on a national scale.

While I was in Oregon, we started to hear rumblings coming up from San Francisco about a new "gay disease." My brother became ill with AIDS and died in 1985. So in the 1980s my focus shifted.

I was working in an alcoholism treatment program in Oregon when I attended a workshop given by Jael Greenleaf, who'd come to train our staff. It was the first time I'd heard the notion of an adult child of an alcoholic and I immediately recognized all the symptoms.

I had an absolutely clear picture of my parents as I was growing up. I realized that in all but one of my relationships, I'd been involved with women who grew up in an alcoholic family, or had themselves had difficulty with alcohol or drugs, and I suddenly understood why I had so thoroughly and personally invested my life work in the field of alcoholism. Soon after that workshop, I started attending support groups for families and adult children of alcoholics.

So I was on my own personal recovery journey and was involved in the early years of the AIDS crisis. I studied and trained with Elisabeth Kübler-Ross, which was quite an experience. I started facilitating her Life, Death, and Transition workshops around the country and integrated her work into my private psychotherapy practice.

Do you have any suggestions about how nongay people can help gay AA members feel welcome in meetings?

I would make most of the same recommendations I made in 1975 at the conclusion of the Fifield Report. One of the most important changes AA members can make has to do with language. If we can incorporate words like "significant other" or "partner," instead of "husband" or "wife," the language becomes more inclusive.

Most important, of course, is to maintain our focus about why people are in AA. They are there to recover. The road to recovery requires honesty and self-inventory, and anything we do that restricts someone's ability to be honest affects their ability to get and stay sober. Thus the answer, as always, lies within. Each of us, gay and nongay, must continually ask ourselves if what we do and say comes from a respectful, loving, and inclusive place.

Chapter 16

Pass It On

Ali M.

[Ali was born in Hato Rey, Puerto Rico. She came into AA in Santa Rosa, California, in 1981.]

I was five when my family left Puerto Rico for France. My dad was in the military. I started drinking in France. In France, they give you wine; wine is part of dinner, and I kind of liked it. I was having a hard time; my babysitter was molesting me, so the wine actually helped me. Then we went to Alabama, and then back to Puerto Rico, then Kentucky. After Kentucky, we went to Alaska. When I was fifteen, we came to Oakland, California. After high school, I lived with my grandparents in Puerto Rico.

I graduated to hard alcohol when we moved to Alabama. In Alabama I was an African American. I wasn't black, but I wasn't considered white, even though I'm light-skinned, because of my Hispanic surname. I was in a lot of trouble through school growing up.

When I came back from Puerto Rico I went to Santa Rosa, and I was using up there. Living in Santa Rosa, it was very country. There were not that many women of color, much less Latinas. I was working at a coffeehouse . . . at the Sonoma County Women's Center, and a lesbian AA group called the Gertrude Stein Group met at the café.

One day I had some friends over, and a police car pulls up, flashing its lights, and they ask for me. "What do you need with her?" [my friends asked.] They said, "We'll tell you when we get to the station," and they handcuffed me and put me in the squad car. *That's it,* I thought. *I can't live my life like this.*

The History of Gay People in Alcoholics Anonymous
Published by The Haworth Press, Inc., 2007. All rights reserved.
doi:10.1300/5699_16

I hated AA. I went to this Gertrude Stein Group because it was close, it was lesbian, and there were women there I knew. I listened to people's stories. There were women at that meeting I hated. I thought they were judgmental, racist, and classist, and, of course, it was my own judgments, right? My own fears.

At the end of the meeting they asked if there were any newcomers, and I raised my hand. "My name is Ali, and I'm an alcoholic, and an addict," I said. Then I just broke down because I'd admitted it— because I'd said it out loud to a group of women I didn't like, to a group of women that didn't really know me, who didn't know my story. They all stood up and clapped.

"We are so glad that you finally came around!"

"What do you mean," I said, "'finally came around'? What are you talking about?"

Well, the café had an office in back where I would sit, smoking my joints, doing my coke, and drinking my beer, but I didn't realize that the smoke was going out under the door into the room where they were trying to hold their meetings.

"This is why we complained," they said, and I felt really bad.

I started going to a meeting at eight [in the morning], to one at noon, and one at eight at night, and I did that for three months. I didn't do ninety [meetings] in ninety [days]; I did about two hundred in sixty days, and it saved my butt. I went with Arial [to meetings], and then with Tam, wherever they went. Then there was the suggestion that I call the Alcoholism Center for Women (ACW) in Los Angeles.

"Here's the number," they said. "Call."

Almost all my friends in the Gertrude Stein Group had been to ACW, and my friend Tam was just awesome. That's something about those women up there in Santa Rosa—"Let's do this thing," they said, so that I can move forward with my life. My roommate drove me down to Los Angeles, and I was at ACW for ninety days. It was one of the best experiences I've ever had. I've got to say that it was just awesome.

The longer I was abstinent and sober, the more feelings and memories came up, [including] a lot of memories about the sexual abuse, which were a lot of the reasons why I used as I used. They came up in therapy, . . . and the first thing I wanted to do was run from the feelings, which is what I'd done all my life. Numbing myself out really helped.

When I said, "I can't do this anymore," and started going to AA, I really didn't have a good grasp of why I was there. At ACW I started understanding why. The counselors at ACW were just amazing and helped me to understand, . . . and it was a big gift that I realized it. My counselor told me that when you do the footwork amazing things happen, and she was right.

It's been twenty-two years, but I can close my eyes and see her in my mind's eye. Barbara B. saved my life. She gave me the tools that I needed. She said, "Do this. This is for you. This isn't for anybody else." And little by little, that wall started breaking down. She started chipping away on it, and then I ended up chipping away at the rest, and I try to do that every day.

I work in the recovery field now. Most of the people I work with are people of color. They have mental health issues and physical health issues and life-threatening diagnoses. They have major disabilities, and they're fragile. They're the people nobody else wants to work with because they are homeless, because they are crack addicts, alcoholics, prison system prostitutes. Most likely, this is their last stop.

I tell them [how AA] works. Although they hate me [when I tell them], I mean, they love me [at the same time] because I don't pull punches. Are they being honest with themselves? Are they being open, and willing to change?

You give service to the ones that need it the most, and if that someone is a homeless addict or an alcoholic that I give my shoulder to, that's why AA was born. That's why AA and NA exist, and it keeps me going today. My clients keep me going today. Working in the field gives me insight into the foundation I'm standing on that's given me twenty-two years of sobriety.

Would you tell me about the Living Miracles conference?

Living Miracles is an AA conference for gay and lesbian people of color, open to all because it's AA. . . . A lot of times people feel, "Well, I'm not a person of color, so I'm not going to go," and what we say is, "You just need to come and support us." It's an AA thing, and you get as much out of it as anybody else.

Living Miracles is like a microversion of a world AA. It's people from all walks of life—Latinas, Asians, African Americans, Native Americans. It's so freeing to me to be there—as a Latina, as a lesbian, as a person who I know is so underserved in the world we live in! We try to provide a safe space where we can say what we need to say to heal.

It is a people-of-color space, but it's really neat to see when somebody will come because they want to see what it's like and want to be a part of it.

If there are white people in a people-of-color (POC) meeting, do you feel, "Well, this was our space, until they came. Now it's not anymore."

No. It is our space, and one of the best parts about it is that we *know* it's our space!

Today I feel comfortable at Living Sober but for many years I did not because there wasn't anybody there like me. There wasn't a space for people of color to talk. Now, with the people who've been making sure there are workshops for people of color, for lesbians of color, for women, it's a feeling of belonging, of owning it, of, "This is mine. This is mine as much as anybody else's."

Today, I take responsibility for having this in my life. It's like going to a meeting and saying, "I'm an addict and an alcoholic." It's about me, not anybody else—my recovery, not yours; my inventory, not yours. The people of color at Living Sober really turned it around for me. That's why I was able to step up to the plate when I was asked to be cochair for POC Living Miracles. You have to be present, for the amount of service you have to do, and for the commitment to your sobriety. And as I was present for other people, I became more present for myself.

Do you know any other people of color with long-term sobriety?

There are one or two I know up there with thirty years, but not a lot. In the Bay Area I know only one.

I feel good being who I am in the world today. And I'm glad that there are more of us that are sober. But out there, it's few and far between. In my community, I am an old-timer because of the length of sobriety I have, and also in age. Most everybody I know in the POC meetings [is] forty [or] under.

I wish there were more of us. If there are twelve people at a POC meeting, that's a good group. It's lonely, I'll tell you. That's what it feels like to me.

Chapter 17

Side by Side in Southern California: Alcoholics Together

Introduction

In 1969, an AA group for gay alcoholics in Los Angeles met for the first time. The six men gathered together that evening chose the name "Alcoholics Together" for their group. Membership in the Alcoholics Together group grew rapidly. Soon there were Alcoholics Together meetings starting in other parts of Los Angeles. Throughout Southern California in the 1970s and 1980s, and in cities as far away as Boston and Toronto, Canada, the words "Alcoholics Together" and its acronym "AT" became synonymous with gay Alcoholics Anonymous (AA).

The Alcoholics Together groups in Southern California used a unique meeting format that included what was known as the "double-anonymity clause." At AT groups the secretary opened the meeting by reading:

> Hello everyone, this is the Wednesday Night AT meeting. My name is ____ and I am an alcoholic and a homosexual. This is a meeting for alcoholics and their gay friends. However, we ask that only alcoholics participate in the discussion. If you do not wish to identify as gay, the secretary will direct you to another meeting.

Following the Serenity Prayer but before "How It Works" was read from Chapter 5 of *Alcoholics Anonymous,* the secretary would read:

The History of Gay People in Alcoholics Anonymous
Published by The Haworth Press, Inc., 2007. All rights reserved.
doi:10.1300/5699_17

As I said before, I am ____, an alcoholic, and a homosexual. We will now go around the room and identify ourselves, starting on my left.

AT's double-anonymity clause would become the focus of much debate in AA.

Jerry B.

[Jerry got sober in 1968.]

There is a saying in AA, "Until we gave up our old ideas, the result was nil," and one of my old ideas was that I couldn't stay sober because I was gay. . . . But finally when I identified with the other gay people who *were* staying sober, I had to give up that old idea.

In 1968, I was going to meetings in San Francisco. I still wasn't out to anybody. This was my little secret. But, apparently, I wasn't keeping it very well, because Don, Gordon, Roland, and some of the others [gay AA members] befriended me.

I talked to them about this horrible secret I was keeping. I'd had five years in AA, and many, many slips, keeping my secret. I believed . . . God wasn't going to help me at all. They convinced me that God would help me stay sober, and that I could be gay and lead a productive life. I was part of the need they saw for a meeting where being gay could be talked about openly. . . .

But the thinking was that I was an example of the gay people who weren't making it in straight AA. *[Laughing]* It's my fantasy to think they said, "Okay, we really need a gay meeting to help this turkey along!" But it was their nurturing, encouragement, and friendship that helped me.

I never thought of myself as self-supporting. I knew that once people found out I was gay I would never be able to advance or participate [in society], yet here [at the Fell Street meeting] were some very successful people. . . . I'm not saying my head was turned by wealth, but that my excuses for not getting sober were no longer valid. *I'm a drunk. I'm a queer. Why should I even try?*

Nobody confronted me. Just by their example they were saying, "Jerry, you're lying to yourself." There was a man at that meeting who ran ____'s first campaign for senator. It wasn't that we became friends, but that he was so visible in his life. I thought, *Wow. Senator* ____ *is where he is today, in part, because of a gay campaign manager.* Those people in the beginning, up on Fell Street, taught me how to be comfortable with myself, and that nothing was wrong with me. I was gay. That was so relieving to me, of what I thought was my burden, or defect, in life.

Some of the regular AA meetings in San Francisco were [attended] by a lot of gay people. . . . These meetings were very integrated; it wasn't the gays on one side and the straights on the other.

How did you know that other gay people were there?

People weren't out in the public sense. When they would speak from the podium, they wouldn't say "my wife" or "my husband." They would say, "My friend" or "My friend living with me." They might say, "My roommate is driving me crazy!" So you'd think, *If it's your roommate, then just move!* . . . And you'd put it together that they were talking about the turmoil of a romantic relationship. The turmoil wasn't because they were gay. It was just the natural course of events, and the solution was to try to work it out through the Steps of AA and Al-Anon.

I arrived in Los Angeles in 1969 and started going to meetings here. Los Angeles has a huge gay population, and the meeting structures were very much the same as they were in San Francisco prior to the start of the Fell Street Group. I met gay people right away.

I hadn't been in Los Angeles long when I saw an advertisement in *The Advocate* that said, "Gay friends of Bill W.? Call this number." A man named Al B. had put it in. A bunch of us called, and we decided that we ought to meet. We met at Troy Perry's house. Troy was starting the Metropolitan Community Church, and we met up in the attic because the living room was being used for services. There were six of us: Al B., Bob G., Jerry H., Jim O., Lee F., and me. . . .

By the second or third meeting, we'd decided to try to list our group in the Los Angeles AA directory, but Central Office wouldn't put the [letter] "G" for "Gay" in the listing, and that presented us with a dilemma. So we decided to call [our group] Alcoholics Together, and to tell the gay people we saw at regular meetings about it, and that's how we spread the word. . . .

The idea was that we would have this thing called Alcoholics Together and attract gay people to meetings. It wasn't to be looked upon as a competing program, but as a funnel. Gay people would be more comfortable meeting with other gay people, and . . . then they'd start going to regular meetings.

We quickly outgrew Troy's attic. I don't think we met there for more than a month because by the third or fourth meeting we just couldn't fit any more [people into the room]. The Mary Lind Foundation offered us a place [to meet], and we moved to their Carondelet Halfway House. Carondelet had a big meeting hall and we filled up two tables in no time. Within a month or two there were thirty to thirty-five people attending on a regular basis. Then [the group] moved to an office building on Hollywood Boulevard, at Sycamore. We rented the room by the month, which allowed us to hold as many meetings as we could. Within six months of our first meeting on [Sycamore], there were 100 to 125 people. And when the women started to come around, it grew even more.

A year after [the six of us] first met, there were easily 200 people in Alcoholics Together, and meetings were starting in other parts of Los Angeles. The word was out, and the [Los Angeles] AA Central Office wanted to know what the hell was going on—what this "AT" thing was.

They elected a man named Don G. to attend our meeting, and it is my understanding that Don went back to the Central Office and said, "There's nothing we can do about this meeting. It is a regular AA meeting. *[Jerry laughs]* And what's more, the fact is that every guy I know in AA was there!" So Don was instrumental in not having AT perceived as a competitive program, and that was very important to me because my loyalties were with AA.

Since the first meeting was a men's stag, by virtue of the fact that it was all men, we decided there ought to be a lesbian meeting. But there weren't enough lesbians to have one, so Bob G. and I became honorary lesbians. We would sit with Marty, and some of the other women, and have a meeting, and it wasn't long before there were enough women to have their own women's stag meeting. *[Laughing]* So that was my only cross-gender experience!

When we moved to Sycamore Street we decided to refurbish the place, and everybody was supposed to come up on Saturday and help.

So Saturday I went over there, and as I'm walking up the stairs, I hear all this hammering, and ripping, and sawing, and I think, *Oh, good. We are really doing it!* And when I got to the top of the stairs I looked into the room. I saw two lesbians, holding a sink out from the wall, while a third one fixed the pipes. And across the room at the window, I see two guys hanging curtains. That was my first introduction to a different culture than the one I'd been dealing with all my life. Growing up on the streets of Brooklyn, then spending six years in the military, then coming out gay, I was in a state of cultural shock.

More AT meetings started to spring up around the city, and [we] began to hear [people] saying things like, "I'm sober one year, and I haven't been to a straight AA meeting." That's how it dawned on us that AT had become a program unto itself or, rather, a structure of meetings unto itself. That wasn't the intent, but AT had now taken on a life of its own. And, people were staying sober. So under the heading of "If it works, don't fix it," that's what happened.

In 1974, the AA General Service Office in New York said they would list gay meetings in the *World Directory* so we would now be included in the book. Then, around 1982, the Los Angeles Central Office agreed to list us, if we became AA groups, so each AT group had to vote on whether to remain an AT group or become a standard meeting; when you identified you would say, "I'm an alcoholic," rather than, "I'm a gay alcoholic."

There was a contingent of people who were very happy being in Alcoholics Together, and now they were being asked to give up their emotional ties to their sobriety, and their original identity. There was a certain level of comfort in being able to say, "I'm a gay alcoholic." But being gay was not viewed as the problem. It could have complicated your alcoholism, but it neither caused it, nor was it the solution. That was always very clear at AT meetings.

The original six of us wanted the meetings to be standard AA with a "G." We never would have had AT if they'd allowed us the "G" in the first place! So we split up, and went to every meeting to give our pitch. We covered them all, from the Valley to Hollywood. We told everyone that . . . we'd never meant for AT to be a competing program. Each group held a vote, and they voted overwhelmingly to rejoin AA, or, I shouldn't say rejoin, but to become standard AA meetings.

Some of our financial processes had to be changed. For example, money from the Seventh Tradition basket would now go to AA, in the standard percentages[1] because, by that time, we had our own published meeting list and our own answering service. The AT Center had to become an Alano Club, as opposed to AT headquarters. And the vote was that this would occur. The Alcoholics Together Alano Club in Los Angeles is still going today. No AT meetings are held there; Alcoholics Together is just the name they gave the Alano Club.

Do you know what prompted the Central Office to start listing gay groups when they did?

I think part of what brought on the change was that the *Los Angeles Times* was going to publish a story about it, and we had to ask them not to do so. We told them we didn't consider it dirty linen, or a hassle, or discrimination, although it probably was. Because we knew that in other cities, like Philadelphia and New York, the Central Offices were listing gay meetings, so it was kind of surprising that Los Angeles wasn't, and we certainly didn't want that as a point of publication. Lee F. talked to the reporter, and it was agreed that we would work it out. Whether the reporter had already talked to Central Office, or if that was the motivation for them to come around, I don't know. But by then, there was a lot of positive publicity about the gay movement. I think they were just waking up and coming to grips with reality. Let me give you an analogy.

When I was growing up, my father was in AA. He was not thrilled with my being gay, and for several years, I was estranged from my family. When I was living in San Francisco, I went to an AA convention in Berkeley, and I brought a friend with me to meet some of my family members, who were also attending the conference. My friend was effeminate, to say the least, and I introduced him around to everyone, saying, "Hi, I'm Ed B.'s son, and this is my friend Norman."

I knew my parents were going to be upset, but I didn't realize how much. My mother and father were taken aback by this boldness, and they communicated that to me. Now fast-forward a few years. I'm living in Los Angeles, and I'm starting to talk to my family again, in a calm and loving way, and one day, I get a phone call from my father. "I want to come down and have lunch with you," he says.

And *[laughing]* after I pick myself up off the floor, I tell him that would be okay. And my father flies down, just to have lunch.

Over lunch he says, "I want you to call your friend Norman and tell him he should run for the [AA] Central Office job I have." At the time, my father was the Northern California representative to the AA General Service Office in New York.

"Norman?" I say. "The guy I introduced you to in Berkeley?"

"Yes."

"What? Are you kidding?"

"No," he says, "I'm not kidding. I want you to tell him. Norm just busts his chops for the program up there." He tells me he's on every committee, et cetera, et cetera. I got tired just listening to how much Norman did.

"Why don't you ask him yourself?" I said.

"I did. He told me he won't do it. He's afraid he won't get elected [because he's gay]." My father had been involved in AA service for a number of years and was widely respected. "If I nominate him, they'll vote," he said.

So I called Norman. I said, "You've got the job, Norman. All that my father has to do is put your name in, and you're elected." But he wouldn't do it. Still, I was taken aback by the turn in my father's thinking: It took maybe six years, but there it was, and that showed me how powerful the program is.

I think a lot of people came around like that. They began to see how serious gay people were about their sobriety, and how hard they worked, doing [AA] service at meetings, at the Central Office, or as general service representatives. My father put himself on the line nominating Norman because there was going to be no mistake once he stood up that Norman was gay!

To see my father change from the terrible person I thought he was, to the open-minded, nurturing person he has become—I always thought my father's mind was set in cement, then reinforced with rebar, with just a little more cement on it, *[laughing]* and I hate that he proved me wrong! But there it is. When I'm struggling with something, I always remember [my father]. I think, *You can change, Jerry. If an attitude is holding you back, you can change.*

I hope I haven't given you the impression that I was any kind of a spearhead in all of these things, as much as I was just going along because, at the time, I was twenty-eight going on fourteen. Once I got to the meetings, I certainly participated on a physical, spiritual, and emotional level, but these were not my creations.

When I was about four years sober, a friend of mine, a roommate, was shot in my backyard. He was selling heroin. I was four years sober, and I wound up in jail. I had nothing to do with it, other than he lived with me, and I was only in jail for a day while the police investigated the shooting. But when I came out of jail, I thought, *Hmm. This isn't the way other AA people spend their afternoons.*

[Laughing] So you see, I really am brilliant! When all else fails, read the directions. I took the Steps, as they were laid out, and my life has changed dramatically. I am employed. I'm a homeowner. I have strong family ties and friendships.

From time to time, you have incidences in your life that tell you why you're sober. When I was a year old, the family put me up for adoption. My father's sister took me in and saved me from the adoption process, and when my mother and father got back together, they brought me to [live with them] in New York. My aunt is now 103, and for the last several years, I have been her caregiver. So the circle is complete. But it couldn't be, if I were drinking. These are the gifts of sobriety.

Joe G.

[Joe got sober in Garden Grove, California.]

A friend of mine who used to be in jail and wrecked-up cars and was in the hospital on a regular basis suddenly stopped doing that.

"What happened to you?" I asked him.

"I've joined Alcoholics Anonymous," he said. I didn't want to hear that.

I was in the construction business, and at the end of every day we'd meet in the big boss's office and have a couple of toddies. After a while I discovered that I couldn't remember getting home. So I stopped doing that, and as a result of not participating in all that drinking, when they rearranged the world, up there at the office, I was on the outside.

I took it as an opportunity to use my health insurance to get some elementary surgery done. "It's a good thing you showed up, Joe," the doctor told me. "We found cancer."

My solution was to drink over it, but then it dawned on me that if I'd been working, I wouldn't have taken the time to go to the doctor, and that by the time I discovered the problem it would have been too late. I realized that, apparently, I had been rescued for something other than getting shitfaced every night. I called my friend.

"What's this AA business about? What happens?"

"We go to meetings," he said. "I'd be glad to take you."

"Oh, no. No, I'll go by myself."

I showed up at my first AA meeting in my three-piece suit, my armor against the world. It was in Garden Grove, in a tiny little room, and the room was full of people. About forty-five, people all dressed very casually, sitting in beanbag chairs smoking seventeen cigarettes apiece.

I don't belong here either, I thought. But they were telling each other all sorts of dreadful things about life, and laughing about it!

And if I didn't immediately accept the fact that I was alcoholic, I accepted that I was as close to being one as I ever wanted to get. They had something I needed, and wanted. So I kept coming back, and I've been coming back ever since, but I left the suit at home.

In 1977, a bunch of us got together. We knew that in Los Angeles they had a thing called Alcoholics Together, and we rented an old after-hours bar, and cleaned it up, and opened it as a place to have gay meetings—where people could talk about problems normal meetings wouldn't accept or tolerate. We formed a nonprofit corporation called Alcoholic Services for Homosexuals, or ASH.

When my friend and I went down to the IRS to apply for nonprofit status, the woman who interviewed us was as nervous as a whore in church. We always went by the name ASH, but our full name was Alcoholic Services for Homosexuals, Inc. So, needless to say, we couldn't disguise who we were or what we were when we were there. I'm sure she expected Sally to be smoking a cigar, and me to be wearing a dress! And we turned out to be just ordinary people.

ASH was in a tiny little shopping center behind a gas station, next to a redneck bar. We were very closeted in those days; at least half our membership entered the building through the back because they didn't want to risk being seen at the front door.

Every now and then, someone would show up at ASH, with a baffled expression, because they remembered the building being an after-hours place. Occasionally, somebody from the bar would show up. He'd see all these queer people, and make a stink, but the police told him, "Leave these people alone."

We made sure we addressed that issue periodically at meetings. "You've got to remember that the police know that we're here," I'd say, "and that we're here under sufferance.[2] So it behooves us not to do anything unethical."

Remember, these were the days of the Briggs Amendment [in California]. There was a lot of ill feeling against homosexuals. If you were queer, you weren't allowed to teach or hold a state job. The police would watch out for us because we were keeping our skirts clean. We were there for legitimate purposes. Nobody was dealing dope, creating riots, scamming on anybody, or doing anything unnecessary. We're sure that, every now and then, an undercover man would show up to attend a meeting, just to make sure we were on the up-and-up. One thing that helped us was that Dr. Max Schneider was on our board. Dr. Schneider is a big name in recovery in Orange County. . . . He had many other things to do, but he would show up once in a while to show that he approved of what we were doing.

How did you find other gay people when you got sober?

Do you mean from the standpoint of cruising or socializing?

Many of the people I've talked with who entered AA in a large city told me they were welcomed by other gay people when they arrived. I suspect that's not the case for everyone.

I don't think I've been to many AA meetings where there wasn't at least one other gay person there. I have two home groups—one gay and one straight—and in my straight group, there are two or three other gay people who show up there, too.

I get my little drum out every now and then, when I hear people talk about only going to gay meetings. I tell them they're doing themselves a disservice. The whole purpose of getting sober is to learn to deal with life! If we treat gay meetings like going to a gay bar, where we do nothing but interact with other gay people, we're not growing. My own example is that I'm an aging, Caucasian male, American, homosexual, democrat, ex-Baptist, et cetera. All of these are different facets of who I am, but if I focus on any one of them, I don't become a whole person.

I don't wear a sign that says I'm a practicing homosexual, but I don't know that it's any secret either. I sponsor more straight men than I do gay ones. I think that's primarily because I'm an old man. I'm nonthreatening. It helps that I've been in a relationship for forty-two years.

Congratulations.

Thank you. When I was arrested for drunk driving, he showed up at the jail at three in the morning to bail me out and said, "I will never do this again, and if you're going to get arrested for drunk driving, do so in Santa Monica. They treat you like a gentleman, and give you a blanket when they put you in the cell." *[Laughing]* So that's good Al-Anon support!

When I got involved with ASH, I was there six days a week. I didn't go on Tuesdays because that was the women's stag night. Like a lot of the other members, I'd go to the Garden Grove Alano Center. I was so used to being at ASH that I went there one day and identified as alcoholic and homosexual, and I almost choked when I said it! But nobody batted an eyelash, and they asked me to lead the meeting the next week. I thought, *You know, I guess this is only a problem in my head.*

In many respects, I get more acceptance as an aging homosexual in a straight meeting than I do at a gay one because of the youth-oriented structure of our community. If you're young and attractive, you're wonderful, but if you're not, you just fade into the wallpaper. It's unfortunate, but that's the way it is.

Have you ever gone to a gay AA Roundup or conference?

The first convention I ever went to was the gay one in Palm Springs in 1978. Up until then, I was ready to throw up every time I heard this "I'm a grateful alcoholic" crap. But on the final day of the conference, 5,000 people held hands and said the Lord's Prayer. Wow, that got me. That was my big moment. I still don't entirely buy the grateful alcoholic line, but I have found that I'm a proud alcoholic.

My gratitude for alcohol is that it finally made me get out of myself. Since I've gotten sober, life has become a tremendous adventure. Recovery has allowed me to be the person I always wanted to be but didn't have balls enough to be. I'm brash enough that I kiss half the men in my straight meeting, too and get away with it! I'm just showing that I love them, and it works. The old me, when I was drinking, wouldn't dare do anything like that.

After announcing in public to a group of strangers six or seven times a week that you're an alcoholic and a homosexual, you get so that it's there. It's just the way things are, instead of, *Shame on me.* This is part of who I am. I've learned not to judge myself by what I think you expect me to be. It's been marvelous, being taught self-acceptance.

Sobriety allowed me to start college at fifty-two. I was working with newcomers at ASH, and somebody said, "Why don't you go to school? You'd be good at it," and I enrolled. I thought I'd become a psych tech and work in a psychiatric hospital. Learning to relate to peers has always been difficult for me, then I got into college, with all these kids. And I'm old enough to be their grandfather! I was treated as an equal—with just a soupçon of deference to the gray hair. The first class I took was anatomy and physiology, and that class was a real eye-opener. On the first test, I didn't see one familiar word. I thought, *Oh god, what have I done to myself?* But I trudged through and went to see my counselor at school.

"What do you want to do?" he asked me, and when I explained it to him, he said, "Have you ever heard of the master's in social work program?" So I finished up at Fullerton College and went down the street to Cal State and continued with Psychology. Then I went to USC, and got my master's in social work, and another one in gerontology. Then I did all the course work for a PhD. I wanted to teach, but at my age, nobody's going to hire me to teach unless I have tons of grant money to pay my salary. And I thought, *I got what I really wanted, which was to get my license, and I'm a therapist. A PhD would have sounded good on a résumé, but what do I need a résumé for? I'm doing what I want to do.*

In 1947, I was in the navy, in Hawaii, and this old lady, who was kind of a mother to the Seventeenth Fleet, adopted me. Seventeen years later, I was in Hawaii on a business trip, and I stopped at the old Army–Navy Y[MCA] for coffee. While I was sitting there, an announcement came over the loudspeaker: "Anyone interested in traveling today, should go see Mrs. L____ at the Activities Desk." I just about fell off the stool! She was still there. And she'd been an old lady seventeen years ago! I went up to see her. "Oh, I know you!" she said, and she kind of adopted me again.

She was at the officers club at least once a month to go dancing till she was ninety-four. She supported herself by playing the piano for an aerobics class, and while she was downtown, she stopped at the old people's home to entertain them, although she was older than any of the residents were.

My sponsor died when she was eighty-four. Her last year she was in senior housing in Denver, on oxygen and a walker, and three days a week, she'd toddle through the lobby, and the old ladies would say, "Elsa, sit down and rest." And she'd say, "I've got all eternity to rest. I've got things to do first." And off she'd go to the food bank to volunteer.

I'm not going to last forever. This is just a short trip we've got here, so each day has got to be somehow meaningful, or I've wasted it. That's what sobriety has done for me. Oh, and that cancer bit, too. That's taking an active interest in life, and that's what I've been trying to do, ever since.

A Conversation with Dr. Max Schneider

Max Schneider is one of the most honored and respected physicians in the addiction field. For thirty years, he was a clinical professor of medicine, psychiatry, and human behavior at the University of California at Irvine. He has served on the federal Food and Drug Administration's Drug Abuse Advisory Committee and the boards of the American Society of Addiction Medicine and the National Council on Alcoholism and Drug Dependence. He is a cofounder and past president of the Southern California Lambda Medical Association.

Dr. Schneider, how did you first come to work with gay and lesbian alcoholics?

I don't know that I made it a specialty. I entered the field in 1953 because, in my fellowship in gastroenterology, I realized that a huge number of the diseases I was learning to be an expert in were due to alcohol: esophagitis, gastritis, peptic ulcer disease, hepatitis, pancreatitis, malabsorption syndrome, esophageal varices, et cetera.

When I opened my practice in Buffalo, I was asked by the now late Dr. Marvin Block if I would cover his practice. Dr. Block was the guru of alcoholism treatment in Buffalo, New York, and chair of the American Medical Association's Committee on Alcoholism. So I got a special education from him. Recovered people had such [a] wonderful outlook on life! My friends had kind of spread the word that I was gay, that I was not a bad doctor, and that I was interested. So that's how it began.

Do you remember meeting physicians who thought that if you cured a patient's homosexuality, that he would no longer be an alcoholic?

Sure. Alcoholism was a disease, but it really didn't become a disease until 1956. Dr. Block was the man who got the American Medical Association to say, "Hey, alcoholism is a disease. It should be treated by doctors in hospitals." And it was very difficult to come out. So nongay physicians didn't know what do with alcoholism, and they didn't know what to do with homosexuals, by and large. Then came Dr. Evelyn Hooker.[3] That was a turning point.

Did you experience homophobic attitudes from other doctors because you worked with gay/lesbian alcoholics?

Not because of my work, but because I was gay. In fact, once word got out that I was interested in gay alcoholics, these doctors were very glad to get rid of those patients and send them to me. As far as negative reactions amongst other doctors, no, except the way that I mentioned. "Go away, gay boy." "Go away, lesbian." "I don't deal with them, but there's a queer doc over there that does." So that was a plus.

In 1970, I became the medical director of a place called Beverly Manor, the first alcohol and drug rehab in Orange County. At that time, I was the only doctor in Orange County that was dealing with alcoholics. I was open [out] to the staff. I've never been very flamboyant—*[Laughing]* Crazy, yes. I have a terrible sense of humor! But an openly gay counselor or physician in the unit made all the difference in the world for gay and lesbian patients. Even today, and I'm just the educational director of the unit, my staff encourages me to touch base with those patients who are gay, lesbian, bisexual, or transgendered to make them feel welcome.

Did you ever meet Marty Mann?

I met Marty around 1970. I was introduced to her by a lesbian doctor who simply said to Marty, as she introduced me, "This is Max. He's a good guy. He's one of us." That was the whole conversation between Marty and me, as far as our sexual orientation was concerned. We just went on and dealt with alcoholism per se. At that time there was another battle going on, the battle of other drug dependency among alcoholics. And there's another battle still going on, and that is the battle of the problem of tobacco addiction.

For the past twenty years, I've been running around the country, screaming, "We've got to treat nicotine dependence the same as we treat other drug addictions! Nicotine dependence is the killer in recovery!"[4] The evidence is very clear. Dr. Hurt at the Mayo Clinic, running the Nicotine Dependence Program up there, and Dr. Janet Bobo, with the Centers for Disease Control in Atlanta, have written substantial papers on the fact that treating nicotine addiction at the same time you treat alcohol and drug addiction is not only helpful, but that people do better when they quit all the drugs at one time.

First treatment centers were saying, "Okay, we'll talk about sexuality as an important issue in treatment." Then came, "Okay, we'll talk about other drugs of addiction in treatment," and hopefully, treatment centers are going to start addressing the nicotine addiction problem. So, inch by inch, we're beginning to say, "Hey, a drug is a drug is a drug; a person is a person is a person."

The fact that I did not become a drug addict or an alcoholic is probably more genetic than anything else. Remember, alcoholism and drug addiction have a strong genetic component, but you can always *learn* to do things! For me, alcohol was not one of them, but smoking was. When I enlisted in the army during World War II—macho, macho, macho—I was introduced to tobacco. I didn't like cigarettes, pipes were laborious, and cigars were absolutely delicious, and as I talk about them now, my mouth starts to water because I became addicted to cigars. I inhaled twelve cigars a day. And what's that got to do with my sexuality? Probably not a damn thing, except that in the 1960s and 1970s, smoking was the thing to do for soldiers, and gays and lesbians, and, certainly, drinking was the thing to do. Addiction to tobacco is much higher among lesbians and gay men than it is among nongays.

Within twenty minutes of smoking a cigarette, you are in withdrawal from the nicotine, and you know that taking another cigarette gets rid of that withdrawal. This crap about "You can't quit everything at once" is pure *el torro caca*. We say we can't do things because we don't know how! That is our ignorance.

That's what bothered me about my early days of dealing with alcoholism. In my early days, I was ignorant. It took a lot of training, and a lot of education, and most of it I got from patients. If you listen to your patients carefully you will learn a hell of a lot.

Although I'm a great advotee [advocate-devotee] of AA, there's a lot of misinformation that can get pushed on the newcomer. One of these is, "You can't quit everything at once." Another is, "Your sexuality has nothing to do with your recovery." The worst is, "Don't take any medications; just work your program." So people go out and shoot themselves because they have major depression or they have bipolar disease. Bill W. was a very open-minded guy. He tried everything. "Let's be friendly with our friends," he said. In other words, be friends with your doctors. Listen to them. Bill would be turning over in his grave today if he heard some of the old-timers say you shouldn't use any medication!

One last question, Dr. Schneider. Have you had any heroes or role models in the treatment field, or in AA?

Oh, yes, and the interesting thing is that some of them are gay. Dr. Maxwell Weissman was one of the great mentors for me; he was an eloquent speaker and a former president of the American Society of Addiction Medicine. The late Drs. Frank Saexas, Ruth Fox, Vernelle Fox, and Jess Bromley were marvelous mentors and leaders in the field. I already mentioned Dr. Marvin Block. And Marty Mann was just absolutely magnificent; she was fearless in her forging ahead for the alcoholic. Among my living mentors are Drs. Melvin Pohl, David Smith, Leclair Bissell, Stanley Gitlow, Joseph Zuska, and Sheila Blum. All these physicians have had great awareness and sensitivity to the special plight of the addicted GLBT population. All of them have led the way to understanding.

Mike K.

[Mike was born in Long Beach, California. He got sober there in 1981.]

I was a wine expert. I founded the Long Beach chapter of Les Amis Du Vin [Friends of Wine]; I wrote a wine column. I took a job working for a wine distributor and my second day I was drunk before I could get in my car to go out on my sales route.

I went to St. Mary's Hospital in Long Beach for treatment [for alcoholism]. I thought that a doctor would give me a pill, that I'd see a psychiatrist who would talk to me, that somebody would do something to me so I wouldn't want to drink anymore, *[laughing]* that if they would just take away my drinking, all my problems would all go away! Poof! So I go into this hospital program, and they tell me I need to go to AA meetings, and write, and work Steps. I thought, *Is this a joke?*

One of the counselors said he'd heard there was a gay meeting at a certain church on Saturday nights and the next night I was at that meeting. I lucked out and got in with a great group. I've been to straight meetings over the years, in different cities across the country and the world, but, generally speaking, they're not a main support of my recovery. I found everything I needed in gay AA.

I understand that at one time you were the executive director of the Van Ness House in Los Angeles, a recovery home for gay alcoholics. Is there anything about gay and lesbian alcoholics, in particular, that you learned while working there?

I learned they all like to get dressed up at Halloween! There's a grand staircase up there, so we always had fun with the costumes. *[More seriously]* Here is something I've learned, being a gay man who has been very sexually active throughout his life.

When I first went to work at the Van Ness House, my biggest fear was that I wasn't going to be able to control that aspect of me, with all these young cute guys coming into treatment all the time—when they are vulnerable, and you are in a position of power. It turned out to be absolutely no problem at all. I realized how ill we are when we get here, how flawed, and the last thing in the world any of us needs is to be taken advantage of, in any way, shape, or form. A good friend taught me that in AA most of the time people want everything for you and nothing from you. That was a whole new way of thinking for me.

I've often wondered whether I would have stayed sober if I hadn't worked in the recovery field; it's a high relapse field. Several people who've worked for me over the years have relapsed, and some never made it back.

I think it was good for me at the Van Ness House. I was responsible for making sure that funding came in, that the plumbing worked, and that there was food on the table. For the first time in my life, I had to put something besides me first. I had to get beyond any personality, including my own, for the good of the facility. The West Hollywood Group, the Silver Lake Group, the Westside Group, and the Santa Monica Beach Group—it took the support of all those groups for the house to be viable. And if the facility wasn't strong, it wasn't going to be there for the people who needed it.

I learned that the people in the gay and lesbian recovering community are human. And that all humans have feelings, and failings. Sooner or later, even the best of them will let you down. There are lots of people here who have nothing that I want, and lots of people who have everything that I want.

Would you talk a little bit about the social model of treatment, the one used at the Van Ness House?

The social model tries not to dwell on the illness of alcoholism per se, for example, that you need medical attention, that you need to be seen by a doctor. It's basically about being observed, and taken care of. It's about one alcoholic helping another. When you're in a hospital, the healing happens between a professional and a client. In the social model, the healing happens between clients. There is no right and wrong here; both things work. I used to describe the social model this way to people who were baffled by this form of recovery: "That which appears least therapeutic is most therapeutic." Like the interaction between the two people who are assigned to cook dinner for twenty others, the need to have somebody assist you, learning that you cannot be so self-sufficient that you can run your life on your own terms. You learn cooperation. You learn to make your bed. Really simple things come together, and make it a healing environment.

Do you have any thoughts on being gay and sober now, compared to being gay and sober when you first came into AA?

Ah, the difference between [being] thirty-two and fifty-two [years old], I guess! Most of my mentors in AA have been older men. Most of them are gone now.

I picked a gay Episcopalian priest to be my first sponsor because I had such a problem with God. I figured, well, how best to challenge that problem! I remember reading the *Twenty Four Hours a Day* book, at my 7:30 a.m. meeting, and I wouldn't even say the word God when it was printed in the book. I just skipped over it. If you'd asked me about it, I would have said it was because I didn't believe in God, but now I would say it was because I was pretty angry with God.

When I moved to Los Angeles, I got a young, attractive sponsor, with a couple of years sobriety, who I knew was going to introduce me to all the right people, and blah, blah, blah *[laughing]* because I still had my motives! I found out that he'd been drinking the whole time he was sponsoring me. But I stayed sober through that, which has led me to wonder whether it really makes any difference who sponsors us as long as we are willing.

Then I heard a man from Scotland speak who had ten years sobriety, and when he spoke I heard my feelings, and he was my sponsor for many years. I owed a lot of money to the IRS, and he said, "Be glad you live in a place where, when a man, or woman, is down they don't kick you, they help you up. The law of your land is there to help you get back on your feet." So I filed bankruptcy, and together, we got through my IRS stuff.

[Mike stops.] He died, five years ago now. Throat cancer—because he couldn't stop smoking, which I could just kill him for! When I was pushing Ensure in a big syringe down a tube into his stomach—

[He falls silent.] He just taught me so much.

I had another sponsor who also died about five years ago. We lived together a while as roommates. When I was working toward my degree, we had to write a lot of papers about family systems. We had to bring everything back to our family of origin. I used to write these papers, and I'd crawl into bed with him and read them to him. He would take me in his arms and tell me, "It'll be alright." *[He weeps.]*

There is something about the wisdom of older people, and the safety. It goes back to having that person in my life who wanted everything for me, and nothing from me. That was unique in my experience. . . .

Ry L.

[Ry got sober in Hollywood, California. Today she lives near Palm Springs, California.]

I was born in New Jersey. One of my older brothers was sort of a movie star, and when I was six, my folks moved out to California because of that. We lived in the Hollywood Hills, just below the sign that, in those days, said Hollywoodland.

There were no gay meetings when I came into AA. There may have been some private ones in people's homes, but I didn't know of any. [Being in AA] was very difficult at the beginning. I felt like, *Yeah, you accept me, and you say you love me, but if you really knew who I was, you wouldn't want me.*

I had a very good sponsor, who knew. I didn't tell her. She just knew, and she said so: "What about the gay issue? Is that a problem for you?" I almost died when she said that!

In 1966, I found a women's meeting at the Radford Clubhouse in North Hollywood, and I finally made friends. If you wanted to find me on a Friday night, you could just call that clubhouse because I was there! The group was about 90 percent lesbian, and we were all getting sober together. Some of us were single, some were with lovers, or we were looking for jobs. We spent holidays together in each other's homes. We became almost like family because none of us had family left.

Like any AA clubhouse, the Radford Clubhouse was privately rented, except that the people who owned it had a caretaker on the grounds at all times. They had AA meetings there from morning till night, and when I was newly sober I spent almost the whole day there.

A lot of the minor people in the movie industry went there—electricians, script girls, maybe a few featured players. . . . Occasionally, there'd be some big recognizable celebrity. The men used to sit in the big meeting room and play cards if there wasn't a meeting going on.

The clubhouse was aware that most of the women in the Friday group were lesbians, and they didn't like it. One night they sent this woman into the meeting, and she started changing the format, and telling us how it was going to be from now on. When we said, "Isn't there supposed to be a group conscience?" she said, "These are the instructions of the clubhouse board. If you want your meeting to continue, you'll have to abide by them."

It was very obvious that they were trying to close the meeting down and to get the lesbians out of there. Some of the women wanted to go to the board and asked if I would go with them, and I said no. "If they want us out of here that bad, then I for one don't want to be here!" and I didn't go anymore after that. They ended the meeting; they took it right out from under us. To this day, I have such a love for that meeting. I still call it the foundation of my sobriety. And when this group of people took it away, for no other reason except that we were gay, I was devastated.

That was the first time I had ever been blatantly discriminated against. With me, I could be anything for anybody, so I was not suspected. The guys at the clubhouse were very good to me, and kind of took me under their wing, but as a group, I know it was very difficult for us. I used to ask my girlfriend, "Do I look butchie?" and she'd say, "Honey, if you had a cigar in your mouth and a carnation in your buttonhole, you would still look like Shirley Temple!"

I was five or six years sober when we began to hear about a gay meeting they were trying to start in Hollywood. At that time, I was going with a woman who was very closeted. We both were. We were executives for a large department store. In that kind of position, you just simply could not—but that's no excuse because we were—except in the AA groups where we felt comfortable—we were closeted everywhere in our lives.

We had objections to this meeting starting up, as a lot of our friends did. "Why are they doing this? Straight meetings got us sober, and they are perfectly fine" was our feeling. "Why separate ourselves again? We've been separated all our lives."

Then some of the people who were trying to get it started spoke to us. They said maybe it was easier for us because we had good jobs, because we lived a closeted life and could get away with it, and things were going well in our lives. But for other gay people, that was not the case. They couldn't seem to get sober in straight meetings. They felt they needed to have a group of their own. And I could see that, and I could understand that because of what had happened with our Friday night meeting. For the first time, I understood how the guys coming off the Boulevard into the program felt [the ones] that were very obvious, because I had always been, like I said, Shirley Temple. I was accepted. I didn't look . . . *[Ry is silent.]*

Because people assumed that you were straight?

I had two little girls. One day when they were very little, I took them to school, I kissed them goodbye in the schoolyard, and when I went back to pick them up after school, they were gone. Their father came and took them, and I didn't see them again until they were grown women.

They were taken away because of my drinking. I was too terrified to do anything about it because I was a lesbian. I was afraid to do anything legally because of what might be said, and then I would lose them permanently.

The women in AA told me I should pray that the best was being done for all concerned, to pray that I would turn out to be the kind of woman I would one day want them to know. I thought it was the best thing because I was such a horrible human being—not only because I was gay but because of my drinking—that they were better off with their father.

In my early years [in AA], a lot of the women who asked me to sponsor them had little children, and it was just gut-wrenching [when my own children were taken away]. It was a very hard time. . . .

My girlfriend and I decided to go to one of the early [gay] meetings. We had to take the elevator up to this meeting, in this big, dark office building, on Hollywood Boulevard. And then, you had to identify not only as an alcoholic, but as being gay! Which was *really*—I mean, I had never said those words out loud to a group of people before! That was really hard to do the first couple of times. But we liked the meeting. We liked the people we met, and we felt comfortable there, surprisingly enough, and we started to attend regularly.

One of the new guys asked me if I would be his sponsor. "Gosh, I don't know," I said. In AA we were always taught that men work with men, and women work with women, so I went to talk it over with my sponsor. That's how upset and confused I was by this! I was so AA that anything AA told me, well, that's what I did, but this was brand new. Everything that was going on was so different from anything I'd been part of in the past, or knew anything about!

"You say this is a gay guy?" my sponsor asked, and I said, "Yes." "So there's no attraction for you? He's not asking you to be his sponsor because he's attracted to you, right?" And I said, "No way!" "Well," she said, "he must really be serious about wanting to stay sober. Why don't you try it?"

So I told him I'd be his sponsor, and from that day to this, no woman has ever asked me to sponsor her. It is a total mystery! Lots of men have. Even today, men ask me to be their sponsor. I've learned so much from sponsoring the guys. I thought we were so different, and I found out that, in emotional ways and spiritual ways, and when we really sat down and talked about what was going on in sexual areas, we were very much alike.

When I was new in AA, I would watch everybody. At the coffee break, everyone seemed to know everyone else. Everyone would be chatting, and hugging, and there I sat. I'm kind of shy. If people want to speak to me, I'm thrilled, but it's difficult for me to speak to someone I don't know. I used to hear people talk from the AA podium who'd say, "The [AA] fellowship is so wonderful. I've got tons of friends for the first time in my life!" And I'd think, *What the hell are they talking about?* I'm not hugging all these people. I'm not experiencing this! Is there something wrong with me, or are they lying? What's going on here?

Then, after a devastating breakup, I moved to the desert. I was going with somebody who wasn't in AA, and I hadn't been to any meetings while we were together, and when we broke up, I was in bad shape. I went to a meeting in Palm Springs, and one of the guys came up to me. I must have looked terrible.

"Are you new?"

"No," I said, and I start feeling embarrassed because I know what his next question is going to be.

"So," he says, "how long are you sober?"

"Oh, about thirty-three years." . . .

"Oh my god!" And we both started laughing.

The community was so welcoming, and so loving. These people loved me back to emotional health, after this horrible breakup, and for the first time I knew what those people in the meetings I went to when I was new were talking about. I was finally experiencing it, for the first time.

I'd been attending meetings here for about a year, when out of the blue I became desperately ill. Something ruptured in my intestinal tract. I was in an ICU unit, and they did not expect me to survive. A gay man took me to the hospital, and [three friends] from the program stayed with me through the entire thing. I would open my eyes, and one of them would be sitting in the corner at all times. They never left me, never.

I remember the nurse coming in and saying, "We have to talk about where you're going to go, when you're released, because you're going to be too sick to go home."

"What do you mean?" I asked her.

"Like a nursing home or a care facility."

Then this voice says, "She's not going to a nursing home."

I didn't know anybody was there, and neither did she, and we both turned around, and this friend of mine from the program was sitting there.

"She's coming home with me, of course," he said. And he took me home and kept me there. I had to escape after three weeks! The care was absolutely incredible. The guys down in Palm Springs are my family. I just love them and they have loved me.

I understand you were on the Van Ness House board of directors in the early 1970s. Would you tell me about that experience?

There was a guy who was very active in [AA] service work, named Lee F. Lee ran the AT hotline for several years and was instrumental in starting the [gay] meetings, and Van Ness House. In 1971 or 1972, he told me they were going to start this recovery home, and that they wanted me on the board.

A bunch of us went over to try to get the place cleaned up before it opened. It was a real dump down on Van Ness Avenue, just below Sunset Boulevard. . . . We were all over there scrubbing the floors and painting. But it was also very exciting because it was the first facility of its kind anywhere. Everyone had their eye on it, to see how it would go.

There were six of us on the board, and I was the only woman. . . . One night we were over at Lee's apartment, hashing out the rules for the house, and it got very late. Lee's boyfriend had already gone to bed. So they said to me, "Will you type these up?"

"I don't type," I said.

They couldn't believe it. "You don't type?"

"No, I don't type."

"That's okay," Lee said. "I'll get my boyfriend to do it."

"Lee!" I said, "You're not going to go wake him up are you?"

"Oh, sure. He won't mind at all." And he went and woke him up, and his boyfriend came out and typed up all the rules. And he wasn't even a member of AA!

At that time, we were partners with the Gay and Lesbian Service Center in Los Angeles, and soon after that, we met with them. They were asking us questions, and Lee, or one of the other guys, would answer, and finally, one of the women from the center said, "I would like to ask my sister a question."

When she said that, I kind of woke up. *Okay,* I thought, *I'm on!* She asked me a question, and I started to answer when Lee interrupted. He finished answering the question, and I deferred to him. She waited until he was finished, and then she said, "Thank you very much for your reply. But now, if you don't mind, I would like to hear what my sister has to say."

And I thought, *Whoa.*

That was a wake-up call—for me, too! I'd never realized the extent to which I deferred to males, even in Alcoholics Anonymous. It had been a pattern of mine since childhood. I have seven older brothers you know!

Have you ever attended a gay AA Roundup?

They used to have a big conference here called the Palm Springs Roundup that was strictly straight. Everybody in Los Angeles AA went to it, and I used to [go] every year. The woman I was with loved to dance, and when the conference had their banquet and dance, we'd go and the gay guys would dance with her. I'd sit and watch or dance with one of the guys. Then, around 1972, somebody decided that we should have our own dance. So we would all go to the convention, and during their dance, we would all be missing; we were out at our own dance! From there, it grew to having dinner together, too, and then it grew to having our own convention. Now the Palm Springs Roundup is gay. The other Palm Springs Roundup has been over for years.

In those days there was a motel down here called the Desert Knight Hotel, owned by two women from the old film industry, in Hollywood, and to stay there, you had to know somebody, or they wouldn't give you a reservation. That way the owners would know you weren't going to tell anyone about who you'd seen. You could be sitting around the pool, and you might see Mary Martin walk by, or Cary Grant, or some of the others [who] might come by to say hello to other gay friends who were staying there.

Is there a lot of long-term sobriety in your AA community in Palm Springs?

Oh, yes. Last year, when I looked at the board where we mark our [AA] birthdays, I realized that every name was double-digit the entire month of October! I don't like to be the center of attention, and every year when it's my birthday, they make a big damn deal. We pass each chip around, to be touched with love by everybody in the room, and they give it to you at the end of the meeting. It's a sharing meeting, and when it's my birthday, every damn person has something to say. Everybody talks about me, and I don't know what to do with myself! I'm just a wreck. So this year, I didn't put my name on the board. I just secretly passed my chip around, and as it went around, someone said, "Oh my god. This chip is for thirty-seven years! Whose is this?" *[She laughs.]* So much for my secret!

One last question for you, Ry. What are some of the ways that being gay and sober is different for you now than it was when you came into AA?

My god. That's such a broad question!

[Laughing] I know. I'm sorry!

[She reflects.] So much of it has to do with the growth I've had in AA, and the age I've gotten to. I'm much more accepting of myself today. As far as I'm concerned, there's no difference between me and anyone else. I don't feel bad about myself for being gay, like I did before coming to AA, and I don't feel bad about myself for being a drunk, like I did when I first came to AA. I feel blessed in both areas in part because I've been able to help so many other people.

I worked in advertising and fashion for years, and I used to think the most wonderful thing would be to work in a profession where you could help other people. I'm an RN now, a psychiatric nurse, and to this day, one of the things that just absolutely blows my mind is that people in AA can help other human beings. We are so privileged to be involved in someone else's life! I don't experience that [anywhere else], even in nursing. I go in to see a patient one day, and the next day the patient is gone. In AA, you are involved in somebody's life process.

My appreciation grows deeper each year. It's just a loving, loving community. I'm sure you'll feel that, and experience it, and I'm very excited for you to come down here and be with us.

Bob G.

[Bob grew up in Ontario, Canada. He got sober in Los Angeles in 1967.]

About six months before I got sober, I started going to the Motion Picture AA Group in Plummer Park, the one the movie stars used to go to. Then New Year's Eve rolled around, and I had a choice of several parties to go to, including one with two friends who always told me I wasn't an alcoholic. I went up there, and that was the start of six months I wish I'd never gone through. I was working in the drapery department at Bullocks department store and missing a lot of work. I'd told everyone that I'd quit drinking, and for the first time, I became a secret drinker. When I returned to AA, they welcomed me back, but I was very upset because they didn't seem to have missed me at all!

I got a good foundation in straight AA. One night I was in the kitchen where they were making coffee before the meeting. I heard a girl say to her friend, "Oh, I know where all the queers go," and my ears just pricked up! She told her friend where they went, and I didn't take long to find out where that meeting was, but it was when we started the gay groups that my whole sobriety changed. I didn't think I had any problems, until I heard them being shared. Then I was able to identify and see that I had some of those fears as well.

We called ourselves Alcoholics Together. Some of the straight members [of AA] were very upset about it, but AT spread so fast, they had to take a look at us! We sent donations to [the General Service Office] in New York once, and they sent them back, saying they couldn't take them because we weren't a part of AA.

In 1974, I left Bullocks and my partner and I opened our drapery shop in Pasadena. "Why don't you start a gay meeting in the shop?" he said. He had started an Al-Anon meeting, you see.

"In the shop? Oh, not in the shop," I told him. "That terrible dump? There are no two chairs that match. It's awful!"

"Start one anyway," he said.

And when we went to the Palm Springs Roundup that year, he went around and told everyone I was having a meeting at the shop on Wednesday, and everyone was coming up to me, saying, "Are you having a gay meeting on Wednesday?" Oh, I was mad!

So on Monday, I had to run around and figure out how to arrange things, like how to put the big tables together. I covered them with red-and-white plastic polka dot cloth. *[Laughing]* After the meetings, we were just about blind!

The shop had a front entrance and a back entrance, and the really anonymous ones came in through the back. People couldn't believe there was a meeting in a drapery shop.

We found that if there was a straight person in the room, everybody sort of clammed up, that people who were having trouble with their homosexuality and their drinking wouldn't talk about it and we finally made it a closed meeting. When somebody new came in who we didn't know, we would walk right up to them and ask if they were gay. We'd say, "This is a gay meeting. You're welcome to stay, but it's not a straight AA meeting. It's a gay AA meeting." And we'd find another meeting for them in the directory, not far from the drapery shop.

That happened a couple of times. It happened with an older couple visiting from the Midwest who'd been sober a long time. They enjoyed our meeting so much they just kept coming to it the whole time they were in California! They enjoyed every minute of it, and, believe me, some of the language was terrible. That four-letter word went around like crazy, you know. I would just cringe.

Apparently, it got back to the Central Office that we were refusing people at the meeting—I heard through the grapevine that some gay person was getting very upset because we were not AA—and they called us to the head office, and we went down. I forget who all was there—Luanne S. and a couple of other straight people. . . . Luanne was all for our meeting. We explained that we weren't throwing people out. We were just making it a closed meeting.

"There's no such thing as a closed meeting," they said.

"Well, you're wrong," I said, "because when women have women's stags, the men don't go."

"Well—they can go. They can!"

"It's the same with us. They can come to our meeting, but we have to tell them it's a gay meeting," I said. "If I walked into a women's meeting, and they told me it was a women's stag meeting, I'd turn around and walk out, unless I was really desperate. And if I thought I was going to drink, well, then I'd damn well stay."

I was a little upset because we were doing everything AA demanded of us. We were sending money to Central Office here, too, and they were taking it, and listing it in the monthly report under "Anonymous Donations."

Then, all of a sudden, I heard that we were going to be listed [in the directory].

I used to have two pitches [a name for the talk one gives when speaking at an AA meeting], a straight one and a gay one. . . . But after I'd been sober a few years, and the gay meetings were well established, when someone asked me to speak, I'd tell them, "They are going to get this the way it is. I am not lying anymore or pulling out this crazy straight story that has nothing to do with [my recovery]." So it worked out—and stopped all the talk about us separating ourselves and labeling ourselves.

The gay meetings started because when a gay person called AA they wouldn't get help. Sometimes they'd be drunk and tell the person [answering the phones] that they were gay. Central Office didn't know whom to call, so we said, "Look, if you get any gay calls, here are some names [of people willing to make a Twelfth Step call to a gay alcoholic]." It depended on who was on the desk, as to how they would handle it. Some people would go overboard to try and find them a gay meeting.

When we got a [Twelfth Step] call late at night, we'd try to find someone to come with us. To me, that's when AA was really interesting and exciting. I thought nothing of going out on a call at three in the morning. People never blamed their alcoholism [for their problems]; they usually blamed their homosexuality. When I would enter, I'd say, "Look, I'm not here to cure your homosexuality, and I don't intend to. I'm here because you've got a drinking problem. Let's take care of that first. We'll worry about your homosexuality later. I'm not drinking, but I'm still gay."

When they were real sick, then they would listen. Hung over and real sick—that's when I liked to get them. And the wet ones [people with the alcoholic dementia of end-stage alcoholism].

They don't do Twelfth Step calls in AA too much anymore. Now an alcoholic can almost walk into any halfway house and get taken in.

Now there are places like Van Ness House and the Alcoholism Center for Women.

Yes, I remember walking up and down off Sunset and Hollywood Boulevard with Lee F., looking for big houses to rent because we were thinking of starting a Twelfth Step house. *[Laughing]* I said to Lee, "Are we going to tell the man or lady what it's for?" and he said, "Let's get the house first, and then we'll tell them!" And we did get a big house. Other than helping to decorate it, I wasn't too involved, but I used to go to meetings there. Van Ness House was a lifesaver.

You mentioned attending the AA Roundup in Palm Springs. Was that a gay Roundup?

For many years, there was a straight Roundup in Palm Springs the first weekend in June. It was jammed. The banquet held 3,000 people! I bought tickets for the banquet and the show a few times. Donald O'Connor was one of our entertainers; Jane Powell was there one year. Fred Waring and his orchestra [played], and they really did it up well. I remember the police chief welcoming us to town: "I just have one request," he said. "Please don't all get drunk at once!"

So this was a big, formal affair!

Oh, yes. This goes back so far that some of the stores still closed for the summer, but once the Roundup started, some of them stayed open because everyone bought new clothes in Palm Springs. The women would wait to buy their evening dresses there.

Then we decided to have our own Roundup. We could only sell 100 tickets, and we did sell them all, honey, and we had our first Roundup, with a dinner and a show, the whole bit! We held it outside, behind the bar called The Tiger. We sold every ticket, and we had a ball. All these lesbians had on long evening gowns, and we were all wishing to try them on! Afterward we went to Oil Can Harry's to dance, and I laughed because the girls had to pull those dresses up over their knees going up the stairs so they wouldn't trip. I heard one of the waitresses say, "I've never seen such a bunch. They're not drinking, but they're tipping like crazy." . . .

Did the people at the other Roundup know about your Roundup?

They knew we were having our own little banquet. They didn't care. They had enough of their own. Of course, there were some old stick-in-the-muds, but most of them were pretty broad-minded, and very supportive. One woman told me, "It's the best thing that ever happened." Montana was terrific. She said, "I was the only one who'll go out on lesbian [Twelfth Step] calls. There are so many gay people dying from alcoholism."

Do you find it harder to get to meetings now that you're older?

I'm home a lot. I'm getting up there, honey! And I don't like to admit it, but some days I feel every bit of it. To be honest with you, I find meetings frustrating. I shouldn't be judgmental, but today I find the younger groups don't seem to take AA as seriously. I'm impatient a little bit that way, but when I get to know the people in the meeting, no matter how young they are, I find out that they are fighting the same battle.

A lot of times I have to push myself out of the house to get to a meeting. Every once in a while, I'll commit to taking the cake every week.[5] The last time I did it out of anger. A few weeks earlier there was someone there with quite a few years of sobriety to take a cake, and all they had for him was a cupcake. A cupcake! With a number on it! And when we had elections a few weeks later, I opened my big mouth.

"I've got a resentment," I said. "Not long ago, we gave a man a cupcake, and I was embarrassed as hell that we would be so chintzy." And it wasn't because we didn't have the money; it was because there's just too much laziness going on. Oh, I was angry! That's one thing I've learned in AA, to speak my mind.

When we first worked with alcoholics, we'd take them to General Hospital. We'd put them on a gurney and roll them into the hallway, and take off like crazy.[6] That's how we'd treat the real sick ones. If they weren't that bad, you brought them home and fed them honey, orange juice, and coffee, pot after pot. You'd read them the Big Book. You'd play it by ear, though, because you could talk your head off, and they wouldn't hear a thing! You'd get them sobered up and hope they'd remember something. Of course, some of them became sponsors to other people.

If it hadn't been for that, I wouldn't be alive today—especially gay AA. I had no trouble with straight AA, but I never found my true story until I was able to get up at a podium and share it as one gay man to another. Some of the younger ones, who've never heard of the drapery shop, or things like that, look at you like they don't know what you're talking about—like when you say that we couldn't dance in bars, or that if two men were caught holding hands, they were arrested.

You could be sober and go to a gay bar and get picked up [by the police]. What do you do when you come out of jail? Do you drink? Do you call your sponsor? Do you learn to handle it?

And there was nowhere else you could go to be with other gay people!

What we used to do, you wouldn't believe it. We would drink coffee like crazy at the meetings, and then maybe ten, or fifteen, of us, would go to a restaurant to eat and talk another couple of hours. I loved to do that. We could talk about anything! It was a good time to get sober. I wouldn't change it for nothin'.

We have come a long way, through patience and persistence. On the straight end of it, the longer they stayed sober, the more tolerant they became. And the longer we stayed sober, the more patient we became. It works both ways, you see. We both grew in our programs. We changed. You can become a completely different person being sober.

Chapter 18

A Few Conclusions
(and Mysteries Solved)

"Did You See Any Gay People?"

One of the things I wanted to learn when I began interviewing gay AA members was how they'd managed to find one another at meetings before the gay groups started. I was surprised to find that my questions on the subject produced a confusing array of responses.

Tony P., George D., and Ruth F., for example, all attended Alcoholics Anonymous (AA) meetings in San Francisco between 1965 and 1969. George, who is gay, and Tony, who is heterosexual, both reported that there'd been lots of gay people at the meetings they attended. They both assured me that everyone was aware of this fact, and quite comfortable with it. However, Ruth said she rarely saw other gay people in AA during that period. She and a group of friends had even conducted an organized search for other lesbians, splitting up and attending different meetings on a given night over a period of several weeks. Comparing their experiences afterward, they found that, with the exception of a single woman, they had seen no lesbians.

Most perplexing of all was this response to my question about whether there were gay people at meetings, which I received from several people. "No," they said, "there were no other gay people at those meetings," and then they'd add, "Except for the really obvious ones."

What? It didn't make sense! And the more people I asked, and the more I thought about it, the murkier the whole business became—until the day I ran across a book by a sociologist named Erving Goffman.

The History of Gay People in Alcoholics Anonymous
Published by The Haworth Press, Inc., 2007. All rights reserved.
doi:10.1300/5699_18

In his 1963 work, *Stigma: Notes on the Management of Spoiled Identity,* Goffman observes that when someone in a group of people has a stigmatized condition that both that individual and the "normal" people around him or her will play a role in "disattending" it (Goffman 1963). It doesn't matter whether it's their homosexuality, their alcoholism, or one of many other possible conditions. For purposes of mutual convenience, both parties will choose not to acknowledge it.

When the stigmatized condition can be successfully hidden, Goffman continues, the task for that individual then becomes one of "information control." As he so eloquently describes the process, "To display or not to display; to tell or not to tell; to let on or not to let on; to lie or not to lie; and in each case, to whom, how, when, and where (Ibid., p. 42)."

Ah. There have *always* been gay people at AA meetings. Sometimes they revealed themselves to the people around them, and sometimes they didn't. Sometimes their signals to one another were received. Sometimes they weren't. Gay people often choose to ignore the gay people they know are present, just as many heterosexuals do. This is often done in an effort to avoid "guilt by association," particularly when it is important to maintain the appearance of heterosexuality.

For example, a gay man who is protecting his heterosexual identity wouldn't want to be seen talking with anyone at a mixed AA meeting who might be perceived as gay. Conversely, the more visible or open a person was about his or her homosexuality, the less likely he or she would be to encounter others who were passing as straight. Under such conditions, it would be nearly impossible for the gay people at a mixed AA meeting to recognize one another.

This dynamic changed dramatically and permanently in the AA community when the gay AA groups began to form. At a gay meeting, people were finally free to interact normally, without hiding, without the secret signals, encoded dialogue, oblique references, and all the other contrivances they were forced to rely on in order to connect with one another in co-occupied heterosexual space.

Several people told me that they'd noticed a dramatic rise in the number of gay people there seemed to be in AA once they began attending a gay AA group. Some of this may be attributed to an influx of new members, but it was more likely the result of the fact that once you had seen someone at a gay meeting, you could recognize and acknowledge each other—from a safe distance, if necessary—in a mixed venue.

What Happened in Los Angeles?

My new understanding of stigma then helped me to solve another puzzle. Why did a parallel AA organization for gay alcoholics develop in Southern California, and why there, but nowhere else in the country?

The development of Alcoholics Together in Los Angeles seemed to defy the forces that shaped the emergence of gay AA groups elsewhere. These included a large gay population, one of the first gay AA groups in the country, and, within a very short period, more gay AA meetings per week than in any other city in the nation at the time. Why did AT develop there?

The answer became clearer as I explored the area's economic and cultural roots, particularly its long and profitable relationship with the film industry.

Hollywood has always gone to great lengths to promote a strictly heterosexual image. In his fascinating book *Behind the Screen: How Gays and Lesbians Shaped Hollywood, 1910-1969,* William Mann documents the complex relationship between the Los Angeles film industry and the many successful gay and lesbian people in its employ—directors, producers, actors and actresses, award-winning writers, composers, set designers, costume designers, makeup artists, and hair stylists, to name a few (Mann 2001).

As homosexual men or women rose to prominence in the industry, the balance of professional influence and social power shifted. The more successful they became, the more the heterosexual people around them were compelled to acknowledge the truth about who they really were. For example, in his conversation with Mann about Hollywood in the 1940s, 1950s, and 1960s, writer/producer Leonard Spigelgass recalled:

Homosexuality in that period had two levels. One, it was held in major contempt and the other, it was the most exclusive club. . . . [I]f you said, "They're homosexual," "Oh, my, isn't that terrible" was the reaction. On the other hand, if you said, "My God, the other night I was at dinner with Cole Porter," the immediate reaction was, "What did he have on? What did he say? Were you at the party? Were you at one of those Sunday brunches?" So you had this awful ambivalence. (Ibid., p. 245)

To a degree unsurpassed anywhere else, the people of Los Angeles have understood the social dictum "Everyone knows, but nobody says." As long as everyone pretended that the gay people in their midst were heterosexual, business in the film industry could continue on as usual. Screenwriter Arthur Laurents recalled:

You could be gay and still be a big success if you kept up the right image. People in the industry just saw this as part of the business—you got married, or you had a lady on your arm at studio functions. It's funny, because after some guy had left with his escort, there'd be all this smirking behind his back. The remarks were made to show they knew the score. It's like they didn't want anyone to think they were fooled. (Ibid., p. 247)

Despite the large gay population in Los Angeles, despite a heterosexual population relatively accustomed to working and socializing with gay people, despite the knowledge that many of the people who wielded power in Hollywood were gay, the pressure to ignore the truth remained high.

So when the members of Alcoholics Together declared that they were sober, *homosexual* members of AA, they broke a very old and very strong cultural tradition in Los Angeles. Who wants to be the first to admit that the emperor isn't wearing any clothes? The unique socioeconomic climate of Southern California was largely responsible for the development of a separate AA service structure for gay people, and it was many years after the founding of AT that this was remedied. The Los Angeles Central Office did not include gay meetings of Alcoholic Anonymous in its schedules until 1982.

On Being Safe, Being Separate, and Being Special in Alcoholics Anonymous

The stress of living with public contempt hurts gay people, and it hurts their families, and concealing one's alcoholism is stressful, even with years of sobriety. Coming to terms with the damage inflicted by addiction and alcoholism is a long and difficult process, one we know must be undertaken in a safe environment, a safe place where people can come to terms with their experiences and heal. At their best, twelve-step meetings provide a unique environment where this can occur, a place where group members are encouraged to talk openly, away from danger, perceived or real, away from anyone they've been threatened by or culturally conditioned to placate and protect.

Still you cannot tell whether people are straight or gay by looking at them. This little fact caused big problems in meetings of Alcoholics Anonymous. It made lots of homophobic AA members uncomfortable to think that there were homosexuals in their meetings. And in gay meetings of AA, how could group members tell whether it was safe to share? Were there straight people in the circle at the meeting, waiting to tell someone they'd been seen at a gay meeting?

The situation is different when a minority's differences are immediately apparent. For example, when a man enters an AA meeting and discovers that it's a group for women alcoholics, he has a choice. He can respect the group's request for separate space and leave, or he can ignore their request and stay. If he elects to stay, his presence will jeopardize its members' feeling of trust and safety. Though his presence may be tolerated, his motives for being there will be suspect, particularly if he continues to attend the group's meetings.

How could the gay members of AA safeguard their groups from people whose explicit intent was to disrupt them? How could they make their groups both accessible and safe, in an era when admitting to homosexuality was grounds for contempt and considered, by some, as an invitation for intimidation and violence?

The members of Alcoholics Together used a simple technique, one that will be familiar to anyone who's heard the phrase "Hello, my name is ____, and I'm an alcoholic." This phrase, when delivered at an AA meeting, turns a shameful confession into a statement of solidarity and strength. To this, the members of AT added "and a homosexual." And with the secretary's request that everyone at an AT meeting make the same declaration, they disarmed anyone who was there with malicious intent in a very effective way. To such a person, stating, "I am a homosexual," in front of the group would be very uncomfortable, yet refusing to do so would quickly make the person's motives clear. From the time of the founding in 1969 to its formal readmittance into the Los Angeles AA service structure thirteen years later, AT served and protected Southern California's gay recovering community. AT's double-anonymity clause ensured that, at their meetings, the floor belonged to the gay members of AA. Many AA members, gay and straight, felt the practice violated AA's Third Tradition. Some saw it as proof that gay groups ought to be excluded from Alcoholics Anonymous. But if AT broke the letter of the law—or, in this case, the Tradition—it upheld the spirit of that law: that every alcoholic has the right to membership in Alcoholics Anonymous.

On Being Special in AA

Many gay alcoholics face a dilemma when they make the decision to attend AA meetings: which is more important—their identity as a gay man or woman in recovery or their need to belong in AA, to fit in, to be "a part of?" Coming out at an AA meeting can be terrifying, but pretending to be someone you're not exacts a price as well. Lying is simultaneously safe and stifling, and it renders gay people invisible in a very fundamental way.

> I'm not going to say very much about myself except that I belong here. Sometimes I have to fight to belong, fight myself to belong—fight that part of me that wants to be so different that I don't belong. Much less often I have had to fight other people in the Fellowship who tell me, in one way or another, that I don't belong.
>
> Nancy T.
> "Gays in AA: Apart of, or Apart From?" (1980)

Because homosexuality is a stigmatized condition that can be hidden, gay people have had to proclaim their difference in order to become visible. They have had to stand up and say, "I *am* different." But in AA there is sometimes a subtle message that thinking you are different from other alcoholics, that being "special," places your sobriety at risk. Where does this come from?

Dr. Harry Tiebout, AA's "first friend in psychiatry," as Bill W. described him, often spoke and wrote about the importance of "ego deflation" in AA. In a 1965 *AA Grapevine* article titled "When the Big 'I' Becomes Nobody," Dr. Tiebout discusses the role of anonymity and ego in sobriety:

> [L]et us take a closer look at this ego which causes trouble. . . . Certain qualities typify this ego, which views itself as special and therefore different.
> . . . Anonymity is a state of mind of great value to the individual in maintaining sobriety. While I recognize its protective function, I feel that any discussion of it would be one-sided if it failed to emphasize the fact that the maintenance of a feeling of anonymity—of a feeling "I am nothing special"—is a basic insurance of humility and so a basic safeguard against further trouble with alcohol. (Tiebout 1965)

AA historian Ernest Kurtz also articulates this view in his book *Not God: A History of Alcoholics Anonymous:*

> AA's unity was rooted in and sprang from its singleness of purpose—helping the alcoholic. Two corollaries flowed from this. . . . [F]irst, Alcoholics Anonymous restricted its endeavors to the one problem shared by all alcoholics—their alcoholism. Second, because all alcoholics shared the problem of alcoholism, any claim to "specialness"—to *difference* from other alcoholics—threatened their sobriety. At depth, as AA's insight of the centrality of the need for the alcoholic to "quit playing God" made clear, it was the claim to specialness that was "the root of [the alcoholic's] troubles." (Kurtz 1991, p. 146)

But you cannot surrender something you haven't got. As the psychologist and Buddhist scholar Jack Engler once observed, "You have to be somebody before you can be nobody." Reclaiming yourself while simultaneously surrendering and admitting your powerlessness is a complex process. Geri C. described it this way: "You have to know yourself, so you can be yourself, so you can get over yourself."

Today, thousands of gay AA members with long-term sobriety stand as proof that gay people in recovery no longer have to choose between being different in AA and being sober in AA.

As long as the stigma of alcoholism and addiction persists, anonymity will protect the members of twelve-step programs. And as long as exploitation, oppression, and alcohol-fueled violence places them in harm's way, the members of AA's many minorities—including women, people of color, the young, and the queer—will need a safe and separate place to meet. As AA has demonstrated so well, it is when an organization makes room for all its members that it becomes truly inclusive, even when they need special time and space apart.

In Closing

To people in AA, the word "sobriety" means a great deal more than not drinking. (A member who's stopped drinking but neglected to apply any of AA's other principles is said to be dry, but not sober.) In a nutshell, sobriety is AA shorthand for "right living." What then can people with many years of sobriety tell us about living a "recovered life"? What has their long practice of AA's Twelve Steps and Traditions revealed to them?

Overall, I found the people I spoke with markedly content. Many of them described struggling at times, as many of us do, with anger, with depression, and with loss, but these struggles took place within the supportive framework of AA. These "long-timers" in AA seemed to hold a broad view of life. They laughed easily. They were quick to forgive. They described, often to their own surprise, the experience of having finally arrived at a place of self-acceptance and peace. They expressed faith in themselves. They expressed trust in others. They expressed faith in the unknown. Many of them spoke of a deep and sustaining relationship with a Higher Power.

Gay people have taken advantage of the opportunity AA has provided to come together in a remarkable way. Many of them have found a spiritual home in twelve-step programs. They have constructed new lives based on honesty, acceptance, and usefulness. They have created a new community with a rich culture and history all its own.

The members of the gay recovering community will continue to play key roles in the fight against addiction and stigma. Daily life with the "double whammy," as Barry L. described it, gives them a unique perspective. "We have been given an extra measure of love," he said, "and from that love, springs a great responsibility." We will need their courage and insight in the long battle against addiction that lies ahead.

Most AA members are well acquainted with the stigma gay people face. The forces that bear down on gay people and their families bear down on alcoholics and their families as well. A great many people will come to know a gay, lesbian, bisexual, or transgendered person for the first time in a twelve-step group.

We have made tremendous progress in our effort to understand and treat addiction. Today we understand so much more about what it means to be gay than we did twenty years ago. We have made great strides in our struggles to secure gay peoples' right to equal treatment under the law. Unfortunately, the fact remains that the most acceptable gathering place for gay people in our culture is still a bar.

But we need not fear alcoholism. History has shown us that recovery always flows around any obstacle fear can throw in its path. In the end, our ability to talk with one another about alcoholism may prove to be our single greatest weapon against it. Born of a slowly fading stigma, the need for anonymity need never prevent the flow of information and hope from going where it needs to go.

Appendix A

The Steps and Traditions of Alcoholics Anonymous

The Twelve Steps of Alcoholics Anonymous

1. We admitted we were powerless over alcohol—that our lives had become unmanageable.
2. Came to believe that a Power greater than ourselves could restore us to sanity.
3. Made a decision to turn our will and our lives over to the care of God, as we understood Him.
4. Made a searching and fearless moral inventory of ourselves.
5. Admitted to God, to ourselves and to another human being the exact nature of our wrongs.
6. Were entirely ready to have God remove all these defects of character.
7. Humbly asked Him to remove our shortcomings.
8. Made a list of all persons we had harmed and became willing to make amends to them all.
9. Made direct amends to such people wherever possible, except when to do so would injure them or others.
10. Continued to take personal inventory and when we were wrong promptly admitted it.
11. Sought through prayer and meditation to improve our conscious contact with God, as we understood Him, praying only for knowledge of His will for us and the power to carry that out.
12. Having had a spiritual awakening as the result of these steps, we tried to carry this message to alcoholics, and to practice these principles in all our affairs.

The History of Gay People in Alcoholics Anonymous
Published by The Haworth Press, Inc., 2007. All rights reserved.
doi:10.1300/5699_19

255

The Twelve Traditions of Alcoholics Anonymous

1. Our common welfare should come first; personal recovery depends upon AA unity.
2. For our group purpose there is but one ultimate authority—a loving God as He may express Himself in our group conscience. Our leaders are but trusted servants; they do not govern.
3. The only requirement for AA membership is a desire to stop drinking.
4. Each group should be autonomous except in matters affecting other groups or AA as a whole.
5. Each group has but one primary purpose—to carry its message to the alcoholic who still suffers.
6. An AA group ought never endorse, finance, or lend the AA name to any related facility or outside enterprise, lest problems of money, property, and prestige divert us from our primary purpose.
7. Every AA group ought to be fully self-supporting, declining outside contributions.
8. Alcoholics Anonymous should remain forever nonprofessional, but our service centers may employ special workers.
9. AA, as such, ought never be organized; but we may create service boards or committees directly responsible to those they serve.
10. Alcoholics Anonymous has no opinion on outside issues; hence, the AA name ought never to be drawn into public controversy.
11. Our public relations policy is based on attraction rather than promotion; we need always maintain personal anonymity at the level of press, radio, and films.
12. Anonymity is the spiritual foundation of all our traditions, ever reminding us to place principles before personalities.

Appendix B

List of Narrators

Narrator	Entered AA in	Years of Sobriety
Ali M.	Santa Rosa, California	21
Mike K.	Long Beach, California	21
Brenda C.	San Francisco, California	24
Geri C.	Portland, Oregon	24
Judy S.	Maywood, Illinois	24
Doug H.	Chapel Hill, North Carolina	25
Joe G.	Garden Grove, California	25
Lee V.	Houston, Texas	25
Moss B.	San Francisco, California	27
Norma J.	Ft. Lauderdale, Florida	26
David C.	Washington DC	28
George M.	New York, New York	28
Kitty M.	New Jersey	28
Nancy T.	Washington DC	30
Sarah G.	New Jersey	31
Blanche M.	Washington DC	32
Jerry B.	San Francisco, California	33
Bob G.	Los Angeles, California	35
Gin B.	San Francisco, California	37

The History of Gay People in Alcoholics Anonymous
Published by The Haworth Press, Inc., 2007. All rights reserved.
doi:10.1300/5699_20

Narrator	Entered AA in	Years of Sobriety
Ruth F.	San Francisco, California	37
Ry L.	Hollywood, California	37
Gordon T.	San Francisco, California	38
Tony P.	San Francisco, California	38
Don K.	San Francisco, California	40
George D.	Los Angeles, California	41
Lois P.	New York, New York	42
L. B.	New York, New York	49
Ben G.	Boston, Massachusetts	50
Pucky	New York, New York	50

Appendix C

Becoming an Ally

If you are a member of a twelve-step program, here are a few suggestions for supporting members in the minority in the meetings you attend.

- Let them know they are welcome, and that AA is a safe place. Say hello. Let newcomers know you're glad they've come.
- Add a Third Tradition statement to your meeting format. For example, "This group welcomes all alcoholics regardless of age, race, sexual preference, creed, or other visible or invisible differences." The NA Preamble reads, "Anyone may join us, regardless of age, race, sexual identity, creed, religion, or lack of religion."
- One Bay Area group added this statement to their format: "This is a Big Book meeting. Readers may, if so inclined, read the text in such a way that is more inclusive of women alcoholics."
- When you share use the phrase "my partner" or "my significant other," rather than "my husband" or "my wife."
- When your area hosts an AA conference for women, or for young people, gay people, or people of color, attend a meeting. When the conferences you go to have workshops for AA members in these minorities, attend one. Show your support. Your experience, and your presence there, will be a healing one.
- If workshops for these alcoholics aren't on the schedule at the AA conference you attend, ask what you can do to make meeting space available. Join the planning committee. Speak to a planning committee member. Put a suggestion in the suggestion box.
- Pass it on.

The History of Gay People in Alcoholics Anonymous
Published by The Haworth Press, Inc., 2007. All rights reserved.
doi:10.1300/5699_21

Here we are. We are all different. We are all pretty special people. But we are also all alcoholics and all sober in AA together. In this, we are more like each other than different. Here in AA, we find the shared humanity that enables us to live out our widely differing lives and pursue our separate and individual destinies. You are welcome to join us.

From *Do You Think You're Different?*

Notes

Preface

1. Two wonderful essays on this topic appear in *The Seductions of Biography,* edited by Mary Rhiel and David Suchoff: John D'Emilio's "Reading the Silences in a Gay Life: The Case of Bayard Rustin," and Blanche Wiesen Cook's "Outing History."

Chapter 1

1. AA groups meet weekly in Canada, England, Australia, Mexico, France, Spain, Austria, Germany, Denmark, Belgium, Sweden, the Netherlands, Iceland, Switzerland, Japan, Ireland, Scotland, Russia, South Africa, and New Zealand.

Chapter 2

1. Copies of Barry's tape are available from the Gopher State Tape Library. You can reach them at 1-877-557-6700 or www.gstl.org. The tape label reads *Barry L., AA, From: New York, NY, At: Gay-Les, Conv. Mpls. Minn., 06/29/85.*

2. For example, in 1977, "Counseling Homosexual Alcoholics: Ten Case Histories," co-authored with Edward Small, Jr., in the *Journal of Studies on Alcohol.*

3. Few AA members alive then, or today, have ever heard Bill Wilson speak. Hearing his voice for the first time and hearing him say something so meaningful must have been overwhelming.

4. Barry's lesbian friend was Marty M. Bill Wilson, who became Marty's sponsor, knew from the beginning of their friendship that she was gay. Giving his talk again the following week in Montreal, Barry remarked that the two older women were among the four who started the *AA Grapevine,* making them either Lois K., Maeve S., or Kay M. Barry's Paris reference suggests that the women had an understanding of homosexuality uncommon in New York at the time, Paris in the 1920s and 1930s being home to a well-known international gay community.

5. For more about this early Boston meeting, read Chapter 4.

6. Barry is referring to Alcoholics Together.

7. AA has two pamphlets in comic book form for people who don't read English well, one for adults and one for teenagers.

The History of Gay People in Alcoholics Anonymous
Published by The Haworth Press, Inc., 2007. All rights reserved.
doi:10.1300/5699_22

8. These references are most likely to Anita Bryant, Jerry Falwell, and California Senator John Briggs.

9. The Multilith draft reads, ". . . Our description of the alcoholic, the chapter to the agnostic, and our personal adventures before and after, have been designed to sell you three pertinent ideas: (a) That you are an alcoholic and cannot manage your own life. (b) That probably no human power can relieve your alcoholism. (c) That God can and will. If you are not convinced on these vital issues, you ought to reread the book to this point or else throw it away" (Dick B., 1998).

Chapter 3

1. The Web site of the National Association for Research and Therapy of Homosexuality (NARTH) states that psychotherapy clients have the right "to develop their heterosexual potential," and that the right "to seek therapy to change one's sexual adaptation should be considered self-evident" (NARTH 2005). In 1997, the American Psychological Association passed a resolution, "reaffirming psychology's opposition to homophobia in treatment and spelling out a client's right to unbiased treatment and self-determination. Any person who enters into therapy to deal with issues of sexual orientation has a right to expect that such therapy would take place in a professionally neutral environment absent of any social bias" (American Psychological Association 1997).

2. An excellent history of eugenics can be found at the online archive of the Cold Spring Harbor Laboratory's Eugenics Record Office, at www.eugenicsarchive.org.

Chapter 4

1. In the early 1950s, the U.S. Post Office established a large surveillance operation targeting homosexual men that included spying, entrapment, and deliberate exposure to cause their arrest. Through subscriptions to pen pal clubs, responses to personal ads, and traces placed on people's mail, the Post Office initiated correspondence with men they believed were gay. Having collected sufficient evidence to generate one arrest, they'd search the victim's mail and initiate correspondence with the men who'd been writing to him to generate more. After nearly fifteen years, the American Civil Liberties Union, in concert with homophile groups such as the Mattachine Society, amassed enough evidence to convince a Michigan Senate committee studying government privacy violations to investigate. The activity finally ceased in 1966 (D'Emilio 1998).

2. In the 1920s, a Lutheran minister from Pennsylvania named Frank Buchman started an evangelical movement called the Oxford Group. Membership in the movement grew through the 1930s. In 1939, the organization changed its name to Moral Re-Armament. AA cofounders Robert Smith and Bill Wilson were both Oxford Group members when they met in 1935. In 1937, Wilson and "the alcoholic squad" in New York separated from the Oxford Group. Smith and the others in Akron followed suit in 1939. Their differences with the Oxford Group included the alcoholic's need for anonymity (versus the Oxford Group's emphasis on public

prominence and promotion), inclusion of the nonbeliever, and the idea that an individual should be allowed to find his or her own definition of God in his or her own time (White 1998; Dick B. 1998).

3. The Lasker Award is the American Public Health Association's award for exceptional achievement in the field of medical research and public health administration. Bill Wilson was nominated in 1951 but declined the honor. Later that year, nonalcoholic trustee and chair of the AA General Service Board, Bernard Smith, accepted the award on behalf of Alcoholics Anonymous as a whole.

4. Felicia G. was the sixth woman to join AA in New York. Her story, "Stars Don't Fall," appears in the second and third editions of *Alcoholics Anonymous*. In it, she describes being sent to Marty M.'s house by Bill Wilson, and being greeted there by Priscilla P., Marty's partner.

5. Bill Wilson's fifteen-year relationship with Helen W. is described in Francis Hartigan's book *Bill W.: A Biography of Alcoholics Anonymous Cofounder Bill Wilson* (Hartigan 2001).

6. The Hetrick-Martin Institute provides services and a safe environment to lesbian, gay, bisexual, transgender, and questioning youth and their families.

7. A sobriety countdown honors the cumulative sobriety of everyone at an AA gathering. As the secretary calls out lengths of time, people stand to be acknowledged by the crowd. Countdowns sometimes end with the newest member, but usually the person with the most sobriety stands last.

8. The relationship between AA and the newly forming National Council on Alcoholism was "the hard anvil of experience" on which several of AA's Traditions were forged (Alcoholics Anonymous 1953; Alcoholics Anonymous 1957; Brown and Brown 2001).

9. In 1934, Ebby T. visited a still-drinking Bill Wilson to tell him about his newfound sobriety and the Oxford Group. Although Ebby was alternately in and out of AA over the years, Bill Wilson always considered him his sponsor. Ebby died sober in 1966. In his remembrance of Ebby in the *AA Grapevine* following his death, Wilson wrote that Ebby "pushed ajar that great gate through which all in AA have since passed to find their freedom" (Wilson 1966).

10. I'd completed several interviews before I realized what a silly and rather impudent question it was to ask, "Were you out?" Of course, being "out" means many different things, depending on the circumstances. Its meaning also changes over time. For example, being out in 1955 would be different from being out in 1975, or 2005, or 2015. What's more, the question always seemed to evoke a sense of remorse and anger in the people I'd asked, as though they felt that they ought to have been more out—more truthful and more courageous—than they had been, regardless of the danger.

11. A great many AA groups never register with the General Service Office in New York (one of a long list of idiosyncrasies that make Alcoholics Anonymous difficult for scientists to measure and quantify).

12. Dr. Elizabeth Blackwell was the first woman awarded an MD degree from an American medical school, in 1849. The American Medical Women's Association awards the Elizabeth Blackwell Medal to women physicians who have made outstanding contributions to the cause of women in the field of medicine.

13. An 1886 compendium of "sexual pathology" by German physician Richard von Krafft-Ebing.

14. Withdrawal from alcohol begins twelve to forty-eight hours after a person stops drinking. Symptoms include nausea, weakness, sweating, and tremor. Some people develop seizures, hallucinate, and hear voices. Left untreated, withdrawals can lead to delirium tremens (the DTs) two to ten days after ingestion of alcohol stops. Symptoms of delirium tremens include anxiety, confusion, sleeplessness, nightmares, fever, disorientation, hallucinations, profound depression, and persistent tremor.

15. This would get a big laugh at an AA meeting because (to their chagrin) the organization, at least in the United States, is so overwhelmingly white.

16. A lay therapist was a person without formal medical training who worked with other alcoholics and was almost always someone also in recovery. The term was coined by Richard Peabody in his 1931 book, *The Common Sense of Drinking,* which was read with great interest by many early AAs. Many of Peabody's ideas, and others from Boston's Emmanuel Movement, would be very familiar to those in AA today.

17. *Cherry Grove, Fire Island: Sixty Years in America's First Gay and Lesbian Town* (Newton 1993).

18. A "father, son, and holy ghost house," more commonly known as a "trinity house," refers to a type of building: a small, three-story rowhouse with a single room on each floor.

Chapter 5

1. The 2002-2003 *World Directory* lists four groups in San Francisco that include the word "gay" in their names. But if you were to check the local directory, which uses codes to indicate the type of meeting that will take place, you'd find seventy-five AA meetings a week for gay people. And of that seventy-five, you'd find two gay meetings for beginners, two for young people, and one conducted in Spanish.

2. Many date the emergence of the modern gay press to June 1969, in the days and months following the Stonewall uprising. Although the first gay publications in America, including the *Mattachine Review, The Ladder,* and *ONE,* appeared in the 1950s and early 1960s, by post-Stonewall standards their circulation was quite limited. Locally circulated bulletins and news sheets could also be found in some gay bars in a few cities before Stonewall.

3. In the 1960s and 1970s, most organizations wanted nothing to do with gay people. As a result, gay groups founded in the 1960s and 1970s, and continuing through the mid-1980s, had difficulty finding a place to meet. The Metropolitan Community Church (MCC), a Christian denomination open to gay people, remains a critical exception to this rule. MCC harbored early gay AA and Al-Anon groups across the United States, particularly in conservative and more rural areas.

Chapter 7

1. It's interesting to note that AA groups based on their members' profession seemed to draw little attention in the debate. I believe this occurred for two reasons: first, because the members of professionally based groups never wanted to have their meetings publicized, and, second, because these groups consisted of men who held positions of significant professional and social authority. Today, contact information for such groups, including the International Advisory Council of Homosexual Men and Women in Alcoholics Anonymous, appears in the *World Directory* under "Special International Contacts."

2. The facts in this timeline are derived from material compiled in the early 1980s by Bob P. and several other AA historians for a book of AA history. The manuscript was requested by AA's General Service Conference but never approved for publication.

3. The Intergroup chair oversees operations of the AA Central Service Office. When John mentions the "Intergroup desk" he is referring to the AA volunteers who answer the phones. Whenever an alcoholic calls for help, they are responsible for finding two AA members who are willing to go talk with the caller about Alcoholics Anonymous.

Chapter 8

1. Bob K.'s story, "On the Move," appears on page 486 in the fourth edition of *Alcoholics Anonymous.*

Chapter 9

1. Randy Shilts' article, "Alcoholism: A Look In-Depth at How a National Menace Is Affecting the Gay Community," appeared in *The Advocate* on February 25, 1976. Shilts later became widely known for his book *And the Band Played On: Politics, People, and the AIDS Epidemic.*

2. The New Group, the first openly gay AA meeting in New York City, was founded in 1972. More of Padric's story appears in the AA pamphlet *Do You Think You're Different?*

Chapter 11

1. Fugitive literature is information outside the publicly available body of literature on a topic, that is, materials other than those published by a government agency, university, or academic press.

Chapter 12

1. The offices of the Society for Individual Rights (SIR), one of San Francisco's early homophile (gay) organizations was at 83 Sixth Street, from 1966 to 1975.

2. Many feminist women entering recovery in the 1970s and 1980s responded to the overwhelmingly male focus of the early AA literature by changing male pronouns to gender-neutral or female ones. For example, in the Twelve Steps, which are read aloud at every AA meeting, the phrase "God, as we understood Him" might be read as "God, as we understood God," or, less frequently, the word God might be read as "Goddess." Today some groups include a short statement in their meeting format to let people know they're free to change the phrasing to make the language more inclusive of women alcoholics (see Appendix C).

3. The Black Cat bar in San Francisco was famous, in both the gay and straight communities, for its drag shows and female impersonators. Pat Bond went on to become a nationally known Bay Area playwright, actress, and activist. Pat died in 1990.

4. In 1972, on the third anniversary of the Stonewall Rebellion, 50,000 people gathered in San Francisco for a march and celebration the organizers called "Christopher Street West." Three years later, in 1976, the parade drew 80,000 people. The following year, 200,000 people attended.

5. In an interview in 1995, Bob H. recalled, "We sent a letter to various gay groups announcing the conference . . . [and to] various Central Offices around the country. Three weeks later we got an anonymous letter, from Texas. In that letter was a check for $3,000. The man said he'd been sober quite a few years, and that he was gay, but that, where he came from, he couldn't be open. He said he thought our idea was wonderful, and here was seed money to help us out."

6. The workshop schedule for the first Living Sober included a "Freewheeling Rap," "Alternatives to Gay Drinking Scenes," "Lesbian Sobriety," and "Sexism, Racism, and Gay Identity in AA." Al-Anon speakers and workshops also appeared on the program, including "Gay Couples," and one called "The Co-Alcoholic."

7. Fort Mason's piers and cavernous warehouses were the primary embarkation point for troops and supplies leaving for the Pacific during World War II.

Chapter 13

1. The other standing committees are Treatment Facilities, Cooperation with the Professional Community, Conference Agenda, Grapevine, Correctional Facilities, Report and Charter, Trustees (nominating committee), and Conference Policy and Admissions.

2. Comparing the draft submitted to the conference in 1983 with the one later approved for publication in 1989, I noted several key differences. One of the most significant was that the collective voice of AA so present in other AA literature, for example, the one that says, "This is how it's worked for us; join us if you will," was missing. Quotes from the stories in the 1983 draft are woven into the pamphlet's narrative and are used to enable a wide range of readers to identify.

Chapter 14

1. Jill Johnston's 1973 book, *Lesbian Nation,* is a collection of political essays and commentary on the lesbian feminist movement. It was especially popular among lesbian separatists and other women on the radical lesbian left.

2. In January 1977, Florida voters passed an ordinance prohibiting discrimination based on sexual orientation. Six months later, following Anita Bryant's "Save Our Children" campaign (slogan: Homosexuals can't reproduce. They must recruit), the ordinance was repealed by a margin of 2-1. News of its defeat galvanized the gay community around the country. In San Francisco, 6,000 people took to the streets in protest. Harvey Milk later credited Anita Bryant with starting a "true national gay movement."

3. AA's 2004 triannual membership survey indicates that 65 percent of AA members are men and 35 percent are women. Those percentages have remained fairly constant for the past several decades, with women comprising between 25 percent and 33 percent of all AA members.

4. "The Promises" can be found in *Alcoholics Anonymous* in the section on Step Nine.

5. "Loners" are AA members who cannot easily get to AA meetings, either because of where they live or where they work (for example, on a ship at sea for many months), or because they are homebound. Since 1974, AA's bulletin, the *Loners-Internationalists Meeting,* has enabled loners to stay connected through correspondence. Today many are active in online meetings.

6. Martin Luther King Jr. was assassinated in Memphis, Tennessee, on April 4, 1968. Eight weeks later, on June 6, Robert Kennedy was assassinated in Los Angeles.

7. "There is a principle which is a bar against all information, which is proof against all arguments and which cannot fail to keep a man in everlasting ignorance—that principle is contempt prior to investigation."

8. After detox, patients were placed in a room designed to look like a bar, complete with dim lights, advertising, and liquor displays. Seated in a comfortable chair they were given a basin, a drug that caused vomiting, and a drink, which they were instructed to consume slowly until they vomited. This procedure was repeated daily with different types of alcohol for ten days.

9. In the New York gay community, the bathhouses were known as "the tubs." In 1968, the Continental Baths opened in the basement of the landmark Ansonia Hotel. During the 1970s, entertainers like Bette Midler, Melba Moore, Cab Calloway, Tiny Tim, and Dick Gregory performed at the Continental Baths, while the audience danced in their towels and cheered from the pool.

Chapter 15

1. The National Institute on Alcohol Abuse and Alcoholism (NIAAA) is charged with creating and administering programs for alcoholism research, education, and

training, and establishing a network of alcoholism prevention and treatment centers. NIAAA was created by the Hughes Act and signed into law in 1970.

2. A tool used to collect and evaluate sociological data, for example, a survey.

3. Shilts' book *And the Band Played On: Politics, People, and the AIDS Epidemic,* was published in 1987. His final work, *Conduct Unbecoming: Lesbians and Gays in the US Military from Vietnam to the Persian Gulf War,* was published shortly before his death in 1994.

Chapter 17

1. Procedures vary, but a common formula for distributing Seventh Tradition donations once group expenses have been met is 60 percent to the local AA service office, 10 percent to AA district and area offices, and 20 percent to the General Service Office in New York.

2. Sufferance is permission given or implied by failure to prohibit.

3. Dr. Evelyn Hooker was the first person to use scientific methods to challenge the prevailing belief among medical professionals that homosexuals were mentally ill. Utilizing standardized psychological tests, and a panel of internationally accepted psychological experts to judge the results, Dr. Hooker unequivocally demonstrated that homosexuals were no more or less pathological than heterosexuals were. She presented her paper, *The Adjustment of the Male Overt Homosexual,* to the American Psychological Association in 1956.

4. Tobacco kills more Americans each year than AIDS, homicide, suicide, car accidents, fire, cocaine, heroin, and alcohol combined, over 430,000 annually. The U.S. Department of Health and Human Services reports that tobacco use, through its influence on heart disease, lung cancer, chronic obstructive pulmonary disease, and numerous other consequences, is America's leading preventable cause of death.

5. Many AA groups celebrate sobriety milestones with a cake. The person with the cake commitment is responsible for bringing a cake on birthday night.

6. Prior to the 1960s and 1970s, before the American Medical Association recognized alcoholism as a disease, most hospitals prohibited the admission of alcoholics. Originally, the phrase "my AA sponsor" referred to the person who'd agreed to pay your bill, if you couldn't, so that you could be admitted to a hospital for detox.

Selected Bibliography

Alcoholics Anonymous (1953). *Twelve Steps and Twelve Traditions.* New York: Alcoholics Anonymous World Services, Inc.

Alcoholics Anonymous (1957). *Alcoholics Anonymous Comes of Age.* New York: Alcoholics Anonymous World Services, Inc.

Alcoholics Anonymous (1976). *Alcoholics Anonymous* (3rd ed.). New York: Alcoholics Anonymous World Services, Inc.

Alcoholics Anonymous (1980). *Dr. Bob and the Good Oldtimers: A Biography, with Recollections of Early AA in the Mid-West.* New York: Alcoholics Anonymous World Services, Inc.

Alcoholics Anonymous (1984). *Pass It On.* New York: Alcoholics Anonymous World Services, Inc.

Alcoholics Anonymous (2000). *A Summary: Advisory Actions of the General Service Conference of Alcoholics Anonymous, 1951-2000.* New York: Alcoholics Anonymous World Services, Inc.

Alcoholics Anonymous (2001). *The AA Service Manual, Combined with Twelve Concepts for World Service, by Bill W.* New York: Alcoholics Anonymous World Services, Inc.

Alcoholics Anonymous (2002). *The AA World Directory, 2002-2003* (three volumes: *Canadian AA Directory, Western United States AA Directory, Eastern United States AA Directory*). New York: Alcoholics Anonymous World Services, Inc.

Alcoholics Anonymous (2003). *Experience, Strength, & Hope: Stories from the First Three Editions of Alcoholics Anonymous.* New York: Alcoholics Anonymous World Services, Inc.

Alcoholics Anonymous (2005). Estimated A.A. membership and group information. www.www.aa.org.

Alcoholics Anonymous 2004 Membership Survey (2005, July). *AA Grapevine,* 62(2).

American Psychological Association (1997). Answers to your questions about sexual orientation and homosexuality. www.apa.org/pubinfo/answers.html.

Anderson, Daniel (1981). *Perspectives on Treatment—The Minnesota Experience.* Center City, MN: Hazelden Educational Materials.

Asbury, Herbert (1933). *The Barbary Coast.* New York: Thunder's Mouth Press.

Beemyn, Brett (ed.) (1997). *Creating a Place for Ourselves: Lesbian, Gay, and Bisexual Community Histories.* New York: Routledge.

A Benediction from Bill (1952, June). *AA Grapevine,* 9(1).

Big Book Facts (2001, December). *AA Grapevine,* 58(7).

The History of Gay People in Alcoholics Anonymous
Published by The Haworth Press, Inc., 2007. All rights reserved.
doi:10.1300/5699_23

Boyd, Nan Alamilla (2003). *Wide-Open Town: A History of Queer San Francisco to 1965.* Berkeley, CA: University of California Press.

Brown, Sally and David Brown (2001). *Mrs. Marty Mann: The First Lady of Alcoholics Anonymous.* MN: Hazelden.

Chauncey, George (1994). *Gay New York: Gender, Urban Culture, and the Making of the Gay Male World, 1890-1940.* New York: Basic Books.

D'Emilio, John (1998). *Sexual Politics, Sexual Communities.* Chicago: University of Chicago Press.

Dick B. (1998). *The Akron Genesis of Alcoholics Anonymous.* Kihei, HI: Paradise Research Publications.

Edelheit, Abraham J., and Hershel Edelheit (1994). *History of the Holocaust: A Handbook and Dictionary.* Boulder, CO: Westview Press.

Epstein, Rob and Jeffery Friedman (2000). *Paragraph 175* [film]. San Francisco: Telling Pictures.

Eugenics Record Office Archive of the Cold Spring Harbor Laboratory. www.eugenicsarchive.org.

Fahrenkrug, Hermann (1991). Alcohol and the state in Nazi Germany, 1933-1945. In Susanna Barrows and Robin Room (eds.). *Drinking: Behavior and Belief in Modern History.* Berkeley, CA: University of California Press.

Finnegan, Dana and Emily McNally (1987). *Dual Identities: Counseling Chemically Dependent Gay Men and Lesbians.* Center City, MN: Hazelden.

Finnegan, Dana and Emily McNally (2002). *Counseling Lesbian, Gay, Bisexual, and Transgender Substance Abusers: Dual Identities.* Binghamton, NY: The Haworth Press.

Goffman, Erving (1963). *Stigma: Notes on the Management of Spoiled Identity.* Old Tappan, NJ: Prentice Hall.

Group Problems and Growing Pains, a Grapevine Milestone Report (1953, May). *AA Grapevine,* 9(12).

Hartigan, Francis (2001). *Bill W.: A Biography of Alcoholics Anonymous Cofounder Bill Wilson.* New York: St. Martin's Press.

Hatterer, Lawrence J. (1970). *Changing Homosexuality in the Male.* Columbus, OH: McGraw-Hill.

Hazelden (2003, Web site). Dan Anderson led social reform movement that humanized the treatment of alcoholics. www.hazelden.org.

How many AAs? (1953, May). *AA Grapevine,* 9(12).

International Advisory Council of Homosexual Men and Women in Alcoholics Anonymous (1982). *1982 World Directory of Gay/Lesbian Groups of Alcoholics Anonymous.* Ann Arbor, MI: IAC.

International Advisory Council of Homosexual Men and Women in Alcoholics Anonymous (1983). *1983 World Directory of Gay/Lesbian Groups of Alcoholics Anonymous.* Ann Arbor, MI: IAC.

International Advisory Council of Homosexual Men and Women in Alcoholics Anonymous (1985). *IAC World Directory: Gay/Lesbian Groups of Alcoholics Anonymous, 1984-85.* Ann Arbor, MI: IAC.

International Advisory Council of Homosexual Men and Women in Alcoholics Anonymous (1987). *World Directory of Gay/Lesbian Groups of Alcoholics Anonymous, 1986-87.* Ann Arbor, MI: IAC.

International Advisory Council of Homosexual Men and Women in Alcoholics Anonymous (1988). *1988 World Directory of Gay/Lesbian Groups of Alcoholics Anonymous.* Ann Arbor, MI: IAC.

International Advisory Council of Homosexual Men and Women in Alcoholics Anonymous (1990). *1990 World Directory of Gay and Lesbian Meetings of Alcoholics Anonymous.* Ann Arbor, MI: IAC.

International Advisory Council of Homosexual Men and Women in Alcoholics Anonymous (1992). *1991-1992 World Directory of Gay and Lesbian Meetings of Alcoholics Anonymous.* Ann Arbor, MI: IAC.

International Advisory Council of Homosexual Men and Women in Alcoholics Anonymous (1998). *1998 International Directory of Meetings.* Ann Arbor, MI: IAC.

International Advisory Council of Homosexual Men and Women in Alcoholics Anonymous (n.d.). *International Directory of Alcoholics Anonymous Meetings for Gay and Lesbian Members* [received 2002]. Ann Arbor, MI: IAC.

Jackson, Joan (1993, September). Communication and culture. *AA Grapevine,* 50(4).

Kennedy, Elizabeth Lapovsky and Madeline D. Davis (1994). *Boots of Leather, Slippers of Gold: The History of a Lesbian Community.* New York: Penguin.

Katz, Jonathan (1976). *Gay American History: Lesbians and Gay Men in the U.S.A.* New York: Avon Books.

Kuhl, Richard (2003). *What Dying People Want.* New York: PublicAffairs Books.

Kurtz, Ernest (1991). *Not God: A History of Alcoholic Anonymous.* MN: Hazelden.

Mann, William (2001). *Behind the Screen: How Gays and Lesbians Shaped Hollywood, 1910-1969.* New York: Penguin Group.

McAdams, Kathleen (n.d.). *The San Francisco Council on Religion and the Homosexual.* www.oasiscalifornia.org/sfcrh.html.

McGarry, Molly and Fred Wasserman (1998). *Becoming Visible: An Illustrated History of Lesbian and Gay Life in Twentieth-Century America.* New York: Penguin Studio.

Mitchell, Alison (1998). "Lott says homosexuality is a sin and compares it to alcoholism." *The New York Times,* June 16, p. A24.

Nancy T. (1979). *Meetings for Gay Recovering Alcoholics, February, 1979.*

National Association for Research and Therapy of Homosexuality (2005). NARTH position statements. www.narth.com.

Newton, Esther (1993). *Cherry Grove, Fire Island: Sixty Years in America's First Gay and Lesbian Town.* Boston, MA: Beacon Press.

Peabody, Richard (1931). *The Common Sense of Drinking.* New York: Atlantic Monthly Press.

Phillips, Thomas (2004). Women: The next frontier for the ex-gay man [review of the book *Changing Homosexuality in the Male*]. National Association for Research and Therapy of Homosexuality Web site: www.narth.com/menus/reviews.html.

Reilly, Philip R. (1991). *The Surgical Solution: A History of Involuntary Steriliza-tion in the United States.* Baltimore, MD: Johns Hopkins University Press.
Rhiel, Mary and David Suchoff (eds.) (1996). *The Seductions of Biography.* New York: Routledge Books.
Shilts, Randy (1976). "Alcoholism: A look in depth at how a national menace is affecting the gay community." *The Advocate,* February 25, pp. 16-25.
S.R.O. for A.A. [news item] (1947, May). *AA Grapevine,* 3(12).
Stryker, Susan and Jim Van Buskirk (1996). *Gay by the Bay: A History of Queer Culture in the San Francisco Bay Area.* San Francisco: Chronicle Books.
Tiebout, Harry (1965, September). When the big "I" becomes nobody. *AA Grape-vine,* 22(4).
United States Congress (1950). *Congressional Record.* 81st Congress, 2nd Session, March 29-April 24, 1950, volume 96, part 4, p. 4527.
White, William L. (1998). *Slaying the Dragon: The History of Addiction Treatment and Recovery in America.* Bloomington, IL: Chestnut Health Systems.
Wilson, Bill (1966, June). In Remembrance of "Ebby." *AA Grapevine,* 23(1).

Audio Recordings

Private collection, transcript of D. R.'s audiotaped interview with Nancy T., November 4, Alexandria, Virginia, 1992.
Fifteenth Anniversary of the Gay Group, Washington DC, December 6, 1986. Cross Junction, VA: Nova Tapes by Earl.
Barry L., AA, from: New York, NY, at: Gay-Les, Conv. Mpls. Minn., 06/29/85, St. Louis Park, MN: Gopher State Tape Library.
Gays Can Stay Sober in AA, Panel discussion, seventh international AA convention, New Orleans, Louisiana, 1980. Dallas, TX: AVW Audio Visual (now AVW-Telav).
Gays in AA: A Part of or Apart From? Panel discussion, seventh international AA convention, New Orleans, Louisiana, 1980. Dallas, TX: AVW Audio Visual (now AVW-Telav).

Index

The History of Gay People in Alcoholics Anonymous
Published by The Haworth Press, Inc., 2007. All rights reserved.
doi:10.1300/5699_24